Solution Focused Practice and Mental Health Crisis

This book provides an interdisciplinary understanding of Solution Focused Practice (SFP) and how to use the approach when working with people in mental health crisis.

The book takes a whole systems perspective, presenting SFP as a "common language" between different professional cultures and making the case for its use across all environments of mental health crisis care. The chapters explore the uniqueness of SFP, chart its history in the UK, and outline ways in which SFP can optimise client agency as well as positively impact worker wellbeing. Anonymised accounts of professional experiences are included throughout to give readers an understanding of how Solution Focused questions can change the balance of power within practice situations and provide inclusive support towards safety and hope.

This will assist a wide range of professionals involved in and working alongside the mental health system including psychiatrists, nurses, social workers, psychologists, therapists, counsellors, and other support staff. We hope it will also be useful for service users.

Nick Perry is a registered social worker, an Approved Mental Health Professional, and is accredited by the UK Association for Solution Focused Practice. He has experience as an educator, supervisor, inspector, and practice lead and is a visiting lecturer at Brighton University.

'Mental health crisis is the daily lived reality of many people in the UK. Navigating our mental health systems can often be experienced as disempowering and dehumanising: a set of difficult hurdles for vulnerable and often stigmatised people. In my experience as a clinician, Solution Focused Practice provides an inclusive and person-centred model for improving the agency, instrumentality, and autonomy of people with mental health problems at points of crisis. Nick and his colleagues are to be commended for bringing together their expertise in this important new book. The book will be of enormous benefit to all practitioners working in crisis environments, and people/communities of colour, based on the clear elucidation of how a Solution Focused approach can support and strengthen anti-racist practice. This is based on the premise that all of society, not just people of colour, thrive when they can find their own solutions to challenges, devoid of the pernicious impact of racism and discrimination.'

Dr Tim Ojo *is a senior consultant psychiatrist in the UK. He is also a qualified coach, leadership mentor, accredited mediator, and organisational consultant with over 12 years of experience in formal medical leadership.*

'There is a consensus that we are facing a crisis in Mental Health care. We need a societal and professional dialogue not just on the causes of this crisis but on what ideas and approaches may offer new ways of helping people who find themselves struggling with a mental health problem. This is particularly so for those who experience the "rough" end of mental health care when they fall into a mental health crisis. *Solution Focused Practice and Mental Health Crisis – Inclusive Support Towards Safety and Hope* looks like exactly the type of book we need to assist in this most vital of tasks. In this book a number of contributors, coming from different professional backgrounds, will outline how Solution Focused Practice can inspire sensitive and creative ways to engage with those in crisis and explain how new directions leading to resolutions are available.'

Dr Sami Timimi *is a Consultant Child and Adolescent Psychiatrist in the NHS in Lincolnshire, UK. He writes from a critical psychiatry perspective and has written widely on subjects related to childhood, psychotherapy, depression, behavioural problems, and cross-cultural psychiatry.*

'Racialised communities may present with various inter-relational, health and socio-economic issues that they may struggle with during experiences of distress. Such issues may require practical solutions and specific knowledge. The use of Solution Focused Practice within the AMHP role (and by other professionals working in crisis environments) invites, with humility and respect, the exploration of issues in a gentle and curious way; that values strengths, unique internal resources; and instils hope. The approach provides opportunities to counteract some of the endemic systemic discrimination experienced in such situations. I hope the book will be read widely.'

Colleen Simon *is currently the Head of Social Work and Social Care for Central and North West London Mental Health Trust, UK. Social worker; lecturer-practitioner on the Bournemouth University AMHP course; she is also an independent trainer.*

'In my career in the UK National Health Service, I have been convinced of the effectiveness of Solution Focused Brief Therapy (SFBT) in benefitting both clients and clinicians to achieve a greater sense of wellbeing and agency in what they do. This is powerfully outlined by the contributors to this book, who come from a wide range of professional disciplines.

'With rising numbers of people needing mental health services there needs to be an approach that provides a common language between the different practitioners involved in their care. I have attended countless multidisciplinary meetings and case conferences in an acute hospital setting which could have been transformed by the Solution Focused approach: where a positive outcome is facilitated through hopeful conversations focusing on the resources of the client, their cultural background, and unique perspective on a better future.

'I believe this book demonstrates that change is happening, and that further possibilities will be generated by the authors' descriptions of SFBT in mental health crisis.'

Kidge Burns *is an experienced Solution Focused practitioner who has worked in the NHS with a variety of clients in different hospital settings. She is also a speech and language therapist; an accreditor for UKASFP; a supervisor; and an experienced author and trainer.*

'This book definitely needed writing. Each chapter addresses a most "frequently asked question" about the Solution Focused approach and does so with convincing examples from everyday practice. It will be a standard reference for practitioners and trainers alike.'

Chris Iveson *worked as a family therapist and social worker before he co-founded – together with Evan George and Harvey Ratner – the BRIEF therapy practice in London. The long-lasting co-operation with Steve de Shazer and Insoo Kim Berg and their many innovations in SFBT has made BRIEF a leading centre for the development and teaching of SF Brief Therapy and Coaching.*

'The application of ideas derived from Solution Focused Practice to mental health acute care is fast gaining ground, and there are many ideas in this publication which have obvious and immediate application. For me, the content about the use of the approach in the Mental Health Act interviewing process is a particularly valuable contribution; and the detailed examples of AMHP practice given by Nick Perry give us a very real picture of these ideas working at first hand. The challenge of applying such an approach where our liberty, as well as our wellbeing is on the line, is well brought out. I recommend the whole publication.'

John Mitchell *has practised as an Approved Mental Health Professional for many years and is an experienced AMHP manager. He is a regular contributor to The Critical AMHP Blog and co-authored the discussion paper: 'MHA Assessments' and s13(1) MHA. His AMHP practice is the subject of Chapter 18 of Horatio Clare's 'Your Journey, Your Way' (Penguin, 2024). Like Horatio, he has experience of being detained under the Mental Health Act.*

Solution Focused Practice and Mental Health Crisis

Inclusive Support Towards Safety and Hope

Edited by Nick Perry

Routledge
Taylor & Francis Group

LONDON AND NEW YORK

Designed cover image: Getty Images

First published 2026
by Routledge
4 Park Square, Milton Park, Abingdon, Oxon OX14 4RN

and by Routledge
605 Third Avenue, New York, NY 10158

Routledge is an imprint of the Taylor & Francis Group, an informa business

© 2026 selection and editorial matter, Nick Perry; individual chapters, the contributors

The right of Nick Perry to be identified as the author of the editorial material, and of the authors for their individual chapters, has been asserted in accordance with sections 77 and 78 of the Copyright, Designs and Patents Act 1988.

British Library Cataloguing-in-Publication Data
A catalogue record for this book is available from the British Library

ISBN: 978-1-032-85648-3 (hbk)
ISBN: 978-1-032-85647-6 (pbk)
ISBN: 978-1-003-51922-5 (ebk)

DOI: 10.4324/9781003519225

Typeset in Times New Roman
by Apex CoVantage, LLC

'When I was younger I used to think that I was very accepting of people, because of my training. I'm realizing that I still have to learn a lot, and to let people be themselves and let go of that idea. If anything, I think I'm still learning to be more accepting of other people as they are. I'm just learning all the time.'

Insoo Kim Berg, in conversation with Victor Yalom
(with the kind permission of www.psychotherapy.net).

Contents

Contributing author biographies

Natasha Adams

Natasha is an innovative, creative, 'can do' thinker who is passionate about celebrating children, young people, and families and bringing voice and participation into all she does. With a Masters in Youth and Community work, Natasha has over 20 years of experience working for local authority, voluntary, and NHS partnerships to develop accessible and innovative services for every child, young person, and family and to facilitate life-changing outcomes. Natasha's experience ranges from targeted outreach projects with young people in the criminal justice system to schools-based interventions, centre-based youth work, and the development of a youth work curriculum for a Surrey youth centre (identified as being one of the most deprived areas in Surrey).

Natasha fell in love with Solution Focused Practice when she joined the team at Learning Space in 2015. Most recently, she has been growing highly successful place-based services and single-session offers to families in the form of a 'triage.' Client and practitioner voices have been central to Natasha's roles as Solution Focused practitioner, manager, training and development lead, and deputy designated safeguard lead.

Natasha has been awarded an Advanced Certificate in Solution Focused Practice by BRIEF in 2022, was accredited by the UKASFP in 2023, and is about to take her experience into private practice.

Aamena Akubat

Aamena currently practices as a clinical research nurse supporting the ASSURED Study: Improving outcomes in patients who self-harm (Adapting and evaluating a brief pSychological inteRvention in Emergency Departments) and SASH Study: Supporting Adolescents with Self-Harm, which are both randomised controlled trials.

She provides Solution Focused therapy to participants who present to Accident and Emergency (A&E) with a mental health crisis as an alternative intervention to those currently available within the NHS. Aamena is keen to better the care and support for people who present to A&E during mental health crises and shape the aftercare following their visit to aid immediate and effective support.

Aamena was previously a psychiatric nurse within a Liaison Psychiatry team based in an A&E department in East London. She also has extensive experience working within a low and medium-secure forensic mental health in-patient setting for adults. During this time, she supported the opening of the first Autism-specialist medium-secure forensic mental health unit in London.

As Aamena continues her journey, she remains driven by a sense of purpose and belief in the power of effective change, with the hope of illuminating a path towards a brighter future for all.

Dr Alexandra E. Bakou

Alexandra E. Bakou is a post-doctoral researcher at City St George's University of London. Alexandra has previously worked as a support worker and team leader in supported housing services for homeless people with mental health needs in London. She has a background in psychology and neurosciences, and she has a particular interest in mechanisms of brief, evidence-based psychological interventions and addiction.

Emma Burns

Emma is a registered psychologist, having worked in mental health, education, and suicide bereavement. She has been employed by New Zealand Police since 2010, discovered the Solution Focused approach in 2011, and has been a self-described 'SF enthusiast' ever since. She spent seven years using the Solution Focused approach working with young offenders before moving into the family harm team in 2018. In 2020, she developed a project, 'Conversations in Custody,' focused on engaging with people in police custody. Emma has now accepted a position as Senior Advisor Organisational Development at Royal New Zealand Police College, where she will contribute to the development of training products and services for NZ Police. This is an exciting step for her, and she hopes to increase the reach of the Solution Focused approach. Emma also has a private business, Connecting with Hope, through which she provides counselling, supervision, and training.

Dr Adam S. Froerer

Adam Froerer, PhD, LMFT, is Director of Research and Training for the Solution Focused Universe (SFU). Adam worked for 11 years as a university professor, where he taught and trained students to be marriage and family therapists and clinical psychologists. After leaving academia, Adam shifted his focus to teaching and training professionals from around the world on how to study and master SFBT. Adam has authored several peer-reviewed journal articles, is the first editor of *Solution Focused Brief Therapy With Client's Managing Trauma,* a book published by Oxford University Press, and an author of *The Solution Focused Brief Therapy Diamond* and *Change Your Questions, Change Your Future,* groundbreaking Solution Focused books published by Hay House, Inc.

Aine Garvey

Aine (Anne) Garvey works for the HSE (the Irish National Health Service) and is also a doctoral scholar at the Centre for Positive Health Sciences at the Royal College of Surgeons (RCSI) in Ireland. Her background is in speech and language therapy and staff coaching. Since first learning about Solution Focused Practice (SFP) over a decade ago, Aine has been practising, training, and researching the benefits of this way of working. The current focus of her research is on the impact of SFP on healthcare workers. Aine is passionate about the potential that SFP has for clients, clinicians, and in organisations generally.

Evan George

Evan is a founding partner of BRIEF, Europe's largest provider of Solution Focused training. BRIEF's work has been presented across most of the UK, and most of Europe, as well as in the USA, Canada, Australia, Singapore, Abu Dhabi, Peru, New Zealand, Japan, and elsewhere. BRIEF has been regarded as one of the most influential teams in the development of the Solution Focused approach. BRIEF's contribution has been recognised in 2012 through the prestigious 'European Brief Therapy Association Distinguished Contributors to Solution Focused Thinking Award.'

With a background in social work and systemic psychotherapy, Evan is the co-author of three books on the Solution Focused approach encompassing the application not only to therapy, *Solution Focused Brief Therapy: 100 Key Points and Techniques* (Routledge) and *Problem to Solution* (BTPress) but also to coaching *Brief Coaching: A solution focused approach* (Routledge). Evan's interests range beyond his work with children, adolescents and adults, couples and families to building co-operation with reluctant clients, leadership, organisational applications of the Solution Focused approach, and conflict management.

Rayya Ghul

Rayya Ghul is an occupational therapist and educator (retired). She was an early adopter of Solution Focused Practice in the UK and a founder member of the United Kingdom Association for Solution Focused Practice. From 1994 to 2000, she worked in Kent across different mental health services and was the approved Solution Focused trainer for the East Kent Community Trust. In 2000, she moved into Occupational Therapy education at Canterbury Christ Church University and developed a Solution Focused Masters courses for health professionals. Rayya supported the establishment of the UK's only fully service user-led mental health service, Take Off. She is the author of two books on Solution Focused Practice, one of which is the first Solution Focused self-help book, *The Power of the Next Small Step,* and a textbook, *Creating Positive Futures: Solution Focused Recovery from Mental Distress.* She was the associate editor of the Journal of Solution Focused Brief Therapy/Journal of Solution Focused Practice until 2023.

Luke Goldie-McSorley

Luke is a passionate and proud social worker and senior practitioner in a Child and Adolescent Mental Health Service in Essex. Prior to this, he spent over 10 years as a social worker in Solution Focused (SF) Edge of Care and Emotional Well-being services in Essex County Council Children's Services. This work supported some of the most high-risk, strained, oppressed, unsafe, and challenging families and circumstances. The success of Luke's work and the incredible work of frontline colleagues in Essex (UK) has inspired small steps of SF revolution in social work and Solution Focused Practice (SFP) across the County.

Luke has a passion for teaching and supporting the development of practitioners working in social care, health, education, charities, youth organisations, and more. He continues to speak at events, train and write about his passion for SFP.

Lauren Jerome

Lauren Jerome is a PhD student at Queen Mary University of London. Her PhD project is exploring the development of a digital tool, based on Solution Focused Brief Therapy, for young people who self-harm. Lauren graduated from the University of Bath in 2016 with a BSc (Hons) in Psychology and has since worked on large, national clinical trials at the London School of Hygiene and Tropical Medicine and Queen Mary University. During her time working at Queen Mary, Lauren conducted and has published a conceptual review and narrative synthesis of Solution Focused (SF) approaches in adult mental health care. Lauren completed her SF training with BRIEF and has undertaken training in therapeutic assessment with SF exits for young people attending A&E following self-harm. For her PhD, Lauren has explored in depth how Solution Focused approaches can be used with individuals who are suicidal and/or self-harm and with children and young people.

Mark Kilbey

Mark Kilbey is Founder and Director of Take Off, the UK's only fully service user-led mental health service. He is a retired Metropolitan police officer who has used his lived experience of bipolar disorder to build a service that offers peer support and meaningful interventions for people with mental health distress. Take Off is unique in providing a peer-led Crisis Group funded by the NHS.

Dr Nektarios Kouvarakis

Dr Nektarios Kouvarakis is a consultant forensic psychiatrist with Sussex Partnership NHS Foundation Trust. He holds an LLM in Mental Health Law, and he regularly works with people in crisis who require assessment under the Mental Health Act 1983 (as amended). He is interested in improving the experience and outcomes for people subjected to compulsory admission and exploring the role of Solution Focused Practice in this effort.

Maria Long

Maria Long is a research fellow at City St George's University of London. She is a mixed methods researcher interested in improving outcomes for young people in distress and their parents/carers. Other research interests include improving social outcomes for people diagnosed with schizophrenia spectrum disorders taking antipsychotic medication. She previously trained as a psychological wellbeing practitioner in a Talking Therapies service.

Professor Rose McCabe

Rose McCabe is Professor of Clinical Communication at City St George's University of London and also Co-Director of the Centre for Mental Health Research. She is an Honorary Professor in East London NHS Foundation Trust, Devon Partnership NHS Trust and Queen Mary, University of London. Her research focuses on micro-analysing communication, understanding patient experience, the therapeutic relationship, and interventions to improve communication, therapeutic relationships, and outcomes of mental healthcare. Central to this work is involving people with lived experience in designing and evaluating new approaches to care. Current programmes of work involve evaluating brief, Solution Focused interventions to support young people and adults presenting to Emergency Departments with self-harm/suicidality in national randomised controlled trials.

Michele Orr

Michele Orr has been a mental health nurse practitioner for the past 13 years with a commitment to Solution Focused Practice and leading Solution Focused teams. She has worked in mental healthcare for more than three decades.

Michele is an experienced clinical supervisor and provides SF supervision to her own teams who work in the Suicide Prevention space. Her own practice is enriched through frequent work in Mental Health Crisis Teams. Michele has been a training provider in Solution Focused Brief Therapy to Psychiatric Registrars undertaking the psychotherapy component of their training, and mental health teams. She has presented at various conferences including the National Suicide Prevention Conference (Australia), National Mental Health Nurse Conference (Australia) and Australasian Solution Focused Association conferences.

Prior to endorsement as a Nurse Practitioner, Michele held senior clinician roles in community Child and Youth Mental Health (rural and metro), including roles in mental health promotion, secondary school nursing, mother and baby and eating disorder units.

Michele holds a Master of Nursing (Nurse Practitioner), Advanced Certificate in Solution Focused Practice (BRIEF) and Level 3 Mastery Certificate in SFBT Diamond Approach (Solution Focused Universe).

Nick Perry (Editor)

Nick is a registered social worker and has been qualified since 2002. He has been practising as an Approved Mental Health Professional (AMHP) continuously since 2007. He has been in a dedicated AMHP and practice educator role for his employing local authority since 2016 and is currently seconded as a practice lead. He has been a visiting lecturer to the Brighton University AMHP training programme since 2020. He was a finalist in the Practitioner-led Research category for the Social Worker of the Year Awards 2024 and has recently been appointed as an Education Quality Assurance inspector for Social Work England.

Nick undertook a foundation training in Systemic Therapy with the Kensington Consultation Centre in 2005. During the pandemic, he was able to undertake the BRIEF online certificate in Solution Focused Practice. He went on to complete the Advanced Certificate in 2022 and became accredited by the UK Association for Solution Focused Practice in 2023.

Guy Shennan

Guy is a Solution Focused practitioner, trainer, and consultant who worked in mental health settings with young people and adults before training as a social worker and working with children and families. He created and co-led the groundbreaking Diploma in Solution Focused Practice at BRIEF before setting up his own consultancy. The second edition of his book, *Solution-Focused Practice: Effective Communication To Facilitate Change*, was published by Bloomsbury in 2019. Guy was the Chair of the British Association of Social Workers from 2014 to 2018, and he is currently engaged in PhD research into the role of hope in social and political activism. He has taught Solution Focused Practice in most of the UK and around the world, including in the USA, Russia, Palestine, Turkey, Mexico, Bolivia, and many countries in Europe.

Foreword

In an era where the world seems to spin faster with every passing day, Solution Focused Practice (SFP) encourages us to take pause – it reminds us that even in the face of complexity, small, purposeful steps forward can create meaningful change. This book invites readers into the dynamic and hopeful world of SFP, a method that puts human strengths and possibilities at the heart of the therapeutic process.

Solution Focused Practice is steeped in optimism, pragmatism, and a deeply respectful belief in the resourcefulness of people. Rather than dwelling on what is broken or dissecting problems to exhaustion, SFP illuminates pathways forward, uncovering the seeds of solutions already present in our lives. It's a methodology that embraces simplicity without sacrificing depth, making it as relevant in clinical settings as it is in everyday conversations.

This book is not just for the seasoned mental health worker or the curious newcomer to the field. Whether you're a clinician, educator, manager, or someone who simply cares deeply about human connection, the principles of SFP will speak to you. You will also see that SFP creates the space for joy, playfulness, and lightness, which can be powerful allies in change.

Nick Perry has led and curated a book that illustrates SFP as a profoundly inclusive practice. It invites people in crisis and mental health workers to co-create a vision for the future that is meaningful to the individual, rooted in their unique experience, culture, and identity. In a world rich with diversity – of thought, background, ability, and aspiration – SFP thrives on celebrating this richness, reflecting a deep commitment to equity and understanding, ensuring that no voice is left unheard.

This book is a much-needed companion for the modern world (particularly so at a time of legislative change here in the UK): the authors have managed the rare feat of crafting a text that is as authoritative as it is accessible, blending academic rigour with the warmth of lived experience.

So, as you turn these pages, prepare to be both challenged and inspired. May you find not only professional tools but also personal insights. Because at its core, Solution Focused Practice is more than a technique, it's a way of seeing the world – and perhaps, a way of living within it.

Dr Sarah Hughes
Chief Executive, Mind

Chapter 1

An introduction and a welcome!

Nick Perry

Thank you so much for picking up this little book!

I am not sure what has drawn you to it – to read this first page – but let me make sure you feel welcomed. I hope that this book will be life-changing for you and for however you are connected to people who experience mental health crises.

The 'why' of the book

The growing of the book has been, in many ways, a journey very similar to my own journey with Solution Focused Practice (SFP): learning how to do something new, from a point of not-knowing, and needing to rely on the expertise of the other people with whom I have had the pleasure of working along the way.

First, I have had to learn how to *do* SFP (and, to a degree, *be* it). Next, I have had to learn how to *apply* it to the role of the Approved Mental Health Practitioner (AMHP), working in England under the Mental Health Act 1983 (as amended), which is my bread and butter.

This AMHP role that I do – a co-ordination role not dissimilar to that of an editor – which is predominantly undertaken by social workers in England and Wales (despite the fact that the training is available to other health professionals, although not doctors) must embody the Guiding Principles of our mental health legislation. We have a core duty to consider (and put in place) the least restrictive way of delivering the mental health care and support that someone in crisis might need (Department of Health, 2015 – due to be amended). We must also involve people in decision-making, empower them and treat them with respect.

For the purposes of this book, we have used UK mental health charity MIND's definition of crisis: 'when you feel at breaking point, and you need urgent help' (MIND, 2020).

Seeing Solution Focused Practice *work* for people who are in crisis is the single motivating force behind the book. Seeing clients begin to visualise (in small steps) the life that they want makes it possible to dream again about a health system – a mental health system – that works; and that is well, in and of itself. A mental health system staffed by people who are skilled to practice in

DOI: 10.4324/9781003519225-1

person-centred ways, skilled-up to support people to reach a place of safety in times of trouble, enabling them to begin to talk about their hopes for themselves and for their families.

In short, I have allowed myself to think about a mental health system led by people from different professional backgrounds who are able to speak a common therapeutic language and who are protected (as far as possible) from burnout. I am profoundly grateful to my co-contributors who have joined me in this ambition and have provided their thoughts and expertise so willingly and so generously.

When this book began its journey, it had as its target audience practitioners from different professional backgrounds who work with people in environments of mental health crisis. These people are still the primary focus for the joint work undertaken here, but as time has gone on, the ambit has expanded to include NHS and local authority leaders, and politicians across the political parties who have a passion for a mental health system that works for everyone – and particularly for people from racialised groups, for whom the statistics of compulsory admission remain worryingly high (Gajwani et al., 2016).

The 'how' of the book

My own journey into the world of Solution Focused Practice has been enabled and impacted by a range of factors.

The Coronavirus pandemic in the UK (and further afield) interacted with various macro- and political processes. The capability and financial security of our National Health Service (NHS) as well as other helping professionals' infrastructure (including local government and the social care sector), was weakened by austerity economics and the political priorities of the Conservative Governments from 2015–2024.

There were implications for our professional practice. Not only did medical hospitals experience chaos during this time, and exhausted, frightened staff try to manage the impact of the pandemic on the general public, but also Approved Mental Health Professionals (and specially-approved psychiatrists – Section 12, Mental Health Act 1983 as amended) continued to be required to assess risk and mental disorder alongside the physical health impact of the virus. This led to a massive spike in my own AMHP workload, a personal fear for my own health and safety, and a real risk of burnout.

As I wrote in the online social work magazine *Community Care* in May 2023: 'My own MHA assessment numbers skyrocketed from 94 assessments in 2019, to 179 in 2020, coming back down to 159 in 2021 and 135 in 2022' (Perry, 2023).

It was this risk of burnout that led me to think about how I might be able to survive professionally when the capability of an AMHP to provide a meaningful, least restrictive option was dwindling at an alarming rate.

I realised that there was still the possibility of using myself as an intervention.

As it happened, this motivation intersected with a rapid moving online of a range of training opportunities (itself an unintended outcome of the pandemic), and with the help of my lovely manager at the time (thank you, Jenny Ryan), I obtained the funding to undertake the BRIEF Online Certificate in Solution Focused Practice with Evan George and Chris Iveson. I went on to complete the Advanced Certificate over the course of 2021 and 2022 (thank you, Barry Davidson, Lynda Casey, and Sara Lewis) and to apply successfully for accreditation with the UK Association for Solution Focused Practice (UKASFP) in 2023.

As soon as the training started in 2021, I began to put it to work within my statutory duties. I made an anonymised record of the situations and client assessments where I used Solution Focused questions. I started to collaborate with others in writing about the application of this way of working to my substantive role (excusing the pun).[1] I also began to think wider than my own tiny part in the whole statutory mental health system in England; I started to wonder what a difference it would make if professionals, in the environments in which we meet people in mental health crisis, were on the same page about how best to help and were able to speak the same workplace language, despite their different qualifying backgrounds . . .

It was this burning thought that led me to reach out to other Solution Focused practitioners and trainers that I had learned with to pull together this book: a book that takes a whole system and multi-disciplinary approach to the work at hand.

It is a key best hope of mine that the book will make it clear to practitioner-readers that applying Solution Focused Practice in mental health crisis work is a choice that we make every day: conversation by conversation; as Guy Shennan will show us, moment by moment. This is a choice borne out of values and core beliefs.

As I have mentioned, alongside this, I have real hope that senior leaders in the NHS and in local government authorities in England and Wales will read the book and be inspired to think about this model for their own workforces. This is for a combination of reasons (including efficiency, person-centred practice, anti-racism, and worker-wellbeing) that will be explored by my co-contributors.

If it is the case that politicians across the political parties, whose duty it is to plan the future of health and social care services in England and Wales, read this book and think both that SFP makes sense and that a step-change is required in the provision of training for the professional disciplines that support people in a mental health crisis, then it will have been a success.

Solution Focused questions look straightforward in themselves – and they are. What is a challenge, and a practice, is to keep asking them, and when you forget to ask them, or you don't ask them well enough, to reflect on it and re-commit to applying the learning at the next opportunity.

I hope you will find encouragement in the chapters of this book to try to apply the questions to your own work, particularly if you are supporting people through such difficulties. I truly believe that there is nothing more empowering, in the midst of a mental health crisis, for someone to hear themselves say for the first time something that might be a first small step towards the future that they want for themselves and the people that they love.

The chapters themselves and their arrangement

In deciding how to lay out the book, it has seemed important, first of all, to underscore the uniqueness of Solution Focused Practice. Of course, there are areas that overlap with other therapeutic modalities, but there are also aspects of SFP that are unique, and I am grateful that Lauren Jerome (building on her previous published work) has demonstrated this so clearly in her chapter.

There is science behind the way that Solution Focused questions are useful to people in crisis, and Adam S. Froerer not only explains the impact on the brain but also shows how Solution Focused questions can be part of the brain's recovery from trauma.

SFP has evolved over the years since its creation by Steve de Shazer, Insoo Kim Berg, and their research team in Milwaukee. In his chapter, Guy Shennan helps us to see how the techniques have become useful in different settings other than therapy, how it can be possible to use Solution Focused questions flexibly and skilfully moment by moment, and how, as a result of this, SFP lends itself beautifully to crisis interventions.

Evan George, one of the three founders of BRIEF, gives us some valuable history regarding the arrival of SFP in the UK and, in his chapter, explores some of the possibilities for its future in mental healthcare services. Rose McCabe and her team at City St George's University of London go on to give an insight into what might be needed in order to train, support, and sustain mental health professionals in this way of working.

Rayya Ghul and Mark Kilbey explain how the approach is not just for mental health professionals – that it is a very good fit with peer support groups and models, empowering service users to support each other towards recovery.

Natasha Adams takes forward the idea of shaping services (for children and adolescents) using the approach. Whilst Luke Goldie-McSorley gives an insight into how the approach can support statutory Children's workers to manage risky situations in a way that co-produces safety.

Of course, despite the changes that are being brought about by the *Right Care, Right Person* debate, the Police will continue to remain first attenders for many people in mental health crises. It is for this reason that Emma Burns brings to us her experience of using Solution Focused Practice with frontline police officers in New Zealand – and the impact that the approach has had on the New Zealand Police as a whole organisation.

Nektarios Kouvarakis, a Greek psychiatrist who has worked in England for over 20 years, gives us an insight into how legislative and policy changes have affected clinical practice. He also explores both the difference SFP could make to the tasks and responsibilities of psychiatrists in different clinical settings, as well as its good fit with amendments to mental health legislation that are to come.

Michele Orr draws on her considerable experience in mental health nursing and managing suicide risk to give a very practical explanation of how to use SFP in high-risk clinical scenarios.

My own chapter documents two case examples in which I use Solution Focused Practice in Mental Health Act work, as well as the way that the approach can support allyship to anti-racist practice.

Last, but not least, Aine Garvey explains some of the potential wellbeing impacts and benefits of SFP for helping professionals and discusses how to embed this way of working into professional practice.

Our 'methodology' and commitment to anti-racist practice

The position of not knowing I have come from regarding the editing of the book has given me some freedom to think about how to pull it together in an authentic way.

The contributors have met online to discuss our personal best hopes for the project, and prior to this, a smaller group of us met to discuss how we would ensure that contributors consider, throughout the chapters, how Solution Focused Practice can support anti-racism.

For those readers who are involved in statutory mental health work in England and Wales, you will already know the extent to which there continues to be a disproportionately high number of people from racialised groups being detained to hospital (Gajwani et al., 2016) as well as placed under supervised community treatment.

Given the imminence of new legislation, we want to address this issue directly and show the way in which Solution Focused Practice can be an ally to anti-racism. We are, of course, aware of the impact that high-profile cases such as Valdo Calocane in Nottingham, England (CQC, 2024) can have on professional efforts to avoid racist processing (Mitchell et al., 2024; Sewell, 2023).

We accept and echo the words of Mo Yee Lee (2003), albeit broadened from only a social work perspective: that Solution Focused Practice

should not be viewed as a panacea or the sole or ultimate solution. Consistent with the philosophy of solution-focused therapy, there is no one solution for any given problem (de Shazer, 1985). Solution-focused therapy, on the other hand, provides a clinical practice orientation – a way of thinking – that is conducive to a perspective of multiple worlds and to strengths-based and empowerment-based social work practice that enables clinicians to participate in a culturally respectful and responsive therapy process with clients from diverse ethno-racial backgrounds.

We came up with the following guidance for the contributors at the beginning of the project:

Please, can you include in your writing any examples of how SF questions uncover new information about resources and capabilities and about the client's network, because the system and the social support and the communities that people are part of are so important . . .

Please, where you can, include practice stories of work with people from different cultural groups, but please don't focus only on the challenges these people encounter. Please focus also on strengths and resilience.

We are not seeking to set up SFP as a 'panacea' . . . SFP could be much more overtly anti-racist as a way of working, but perhaps the baked-in 'not knowing' can promote questions which result in answers that are surprising, and can challenge assumptions, prejudice, stereotypes?

Ultimately, what we're really looking for is to be able to show how SFP really uncovers these alternative stories of strength and resourcefulness.

I hope that you enjoy the book and that you find it useful, that it will be the kind of book you will keep in your work bag to dip into between visits, and that – if you do find it useful – you will share it with your colleagues.

Note

1   Under s13(1) of the Mental Health Act (1983), as amended, AMHPs need to consider, on behalf of their local authority, whether an *application* for detention to hospital is required, given the client's circumstances.

References

Care Quality Commission. (2024). *Special review of mental health services at Nottinghamshire Healthcare NHS Foundation Trust: Part 2*. Care Quality Commission. (cqc.org.uk).

de Shazer, S. (1985). *Keys to solutions in brief therapy*. W. W. Norton.

Department of Health. (2015). *Mental Health Act 1983: Code of practice*. The Stationery Office. GOV.UK (www.gov.uk).

Department of Health & Social Care. (2018). *Modernising the Mental Health Act – Increasing choice, reducing compulsion. Final report of the Independent Review of the Mental Health Act 1983*. (publishing.service.gov.uk).

Gajwani, R., Parsons, H., Birchwood, M., & Singh, S. (2016). Ethnicity and detention: Are Black and minority ethnic (BME) groups disproportionately detained under the Mental Health Act 2007? *Soc Psychiatry Psychiatr Epidemiol, 51*, 703–711.

Lee, M. Y. (2003). A solution-focused approach to cross-cultural clinical social work practice: Utilizing cultural strengths. *Families in Society, 84*(3). https://doi.org/10.1606/1044-3894.118.

Mental Health Act. (1983). *Mental Health Act 1983*. (legislation.gov.uk).

MIND. (2020). *Crisis services and planning*. Retrieved August 27, 2024, from www.mind.org.uk/information-support/guides-to-support-and-services/crisis-services/#:~:text=What's%20a%20mental%20health%20crisis,%2C%20or%20feeling%20very%20paranoid).

Mitchell, J., Lewis, R., & Simpson, M. (2024). *MHA assessments and s13(1) MHA 1983: 'New' AMHP practices within existing law*. AMHP Leads Network – Resources Page (padlet.com).

Perry, N. (2023, May). *Give AMHPs the therapeutic tools that they need to underpin least restrictive practice*. Community Care. www.communitycare.co.uk.

Sewell, H. (2023). Mental health act assessments: No Trace of Race. The role of the AMHP in anti-racist practice. Blog Home. www.the-critical-amhp.com.

Chapter 2

The uniqueness of Solution Focused Practice

Lauren Jerome

The notion of 'Brief Therapy' was first introduced by Watzlawick et al., 1974. They described a therapeutic approach with the main premise that the need to understand the cause of a problem is not required. Instead, how the problem manifests in the present is the focus of therapy. How the problem is maintained through attempts to solve it is explored, and small goals are established. A plan to implement the change should be decided upon, and if this does not bring about the desired change: try something else.

This model of therapy was further developed and called 'Solution-Focused Brief Therapy' (SFBT) in the 1980s by Steve de Shazer and colleagues. They began with the idea of searching for what therapists do in a session that 'works', in order to encourage them to do more of it. This idea encompassed both the therapist and the clients, with the underlying premise being: 'If it works, do more of it. If it doesn't work, don't do it again; do something else' (de Shazer et al., 1986). de Shazer suggested four key, recognisable characteristics of SFBT: first, asking the miracle question; second, at least once, the client is asked to rate something on a scale; third, at some point, the therapist takes a break; and fourth, after the break, the therapist provides the client with a compliment, often followed by a suggestion or homework task.

SFBT has developed and evolved since then. Gingerich and Peterson (2013) add to de Shazer's characteristics by suggesting there are six key components of SFBT, including specific goals, the miracle question, scaling questions, searching for exceptions, compliments, and homework.

For the purposes of this book, we have begun to talk about Solution Focused Practice – as opposed to SFBT – because the approach is increasingly being used by professionals (and in settings) who may not describe their work as therapy.

To help conceptualise more recent understandings of Solution Focused approaches, Jerome et al. (2023) developed a conceptual framework based on a systematic search of the literature for approaches described as 'solution-focused' delivered in the context of adult mental health research.

Although this framework is based on Solution Focused work in adult mental health contexts specifically, it provides a framework of components we can consider applying more broadly to individuals in crisis.

DOI: 10.4324/9781003519225-2

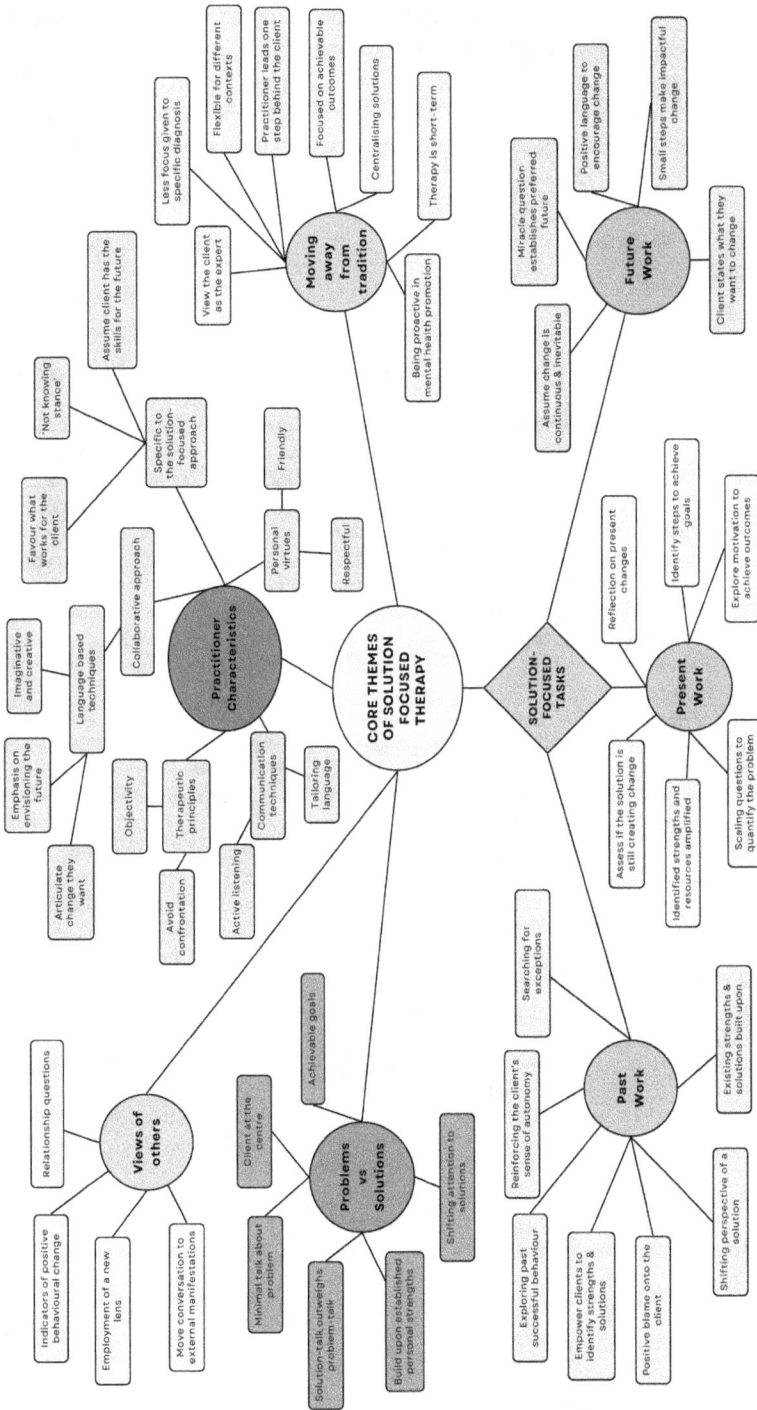

Figure 2.1 Conceptual framework for solution-focused approaches described in the adult mental health literature (Jerome et al. (2023). Solution-focused approaches in adult mental health research: A conceptual literature review and narrative synthesis [Review]. Frontiers in Psychiatry, 14. https://doi.org/10.3389/fpsyt.2023.1068006).

Sixteen different components to Solution Focused approaches were identified, and a conceptual map of the approach was developed (see Figure 2.1) encompassing its move away from traditional approaches, key practitioner characteristics, the views of others used in the approach, the tension of problems versus solutions, and specific Solution Focused tasks including work focused on the past, present, and future.

As part of this work, they also considered the Waltz et al. (1993) model for treatment distinctiveness, summarising what seemed to make Solution Focused approaches

Table 2.1 Essential and unique components of Solution Focused approaches, Cognitive Behavioural Therapy (CBT), and Psychodynamic Therapy. Solution Focused reprinted from Jerome et al. (2023). CBT reprinted from Clinical Psychology Review, 22, Blagys & Hilsenroth, Distinctive activities of cognitive–behavioral therapy; A review of the comparative psychotherapy process literature, 671–706, Copyright (2002), with permission from Elsevier. Psychodynamic reprinted from Clinical Psychology: Science and Practice, 7(2), Blagys & Hilsenroth, Distinctive Features of Short-Term Psychodynamic-Interpersonal Psychotherapy: A Review of the Comparative Psychotherapy Process Literature, 167–188, Table 8. Summary of distinctive features of psychodynamic-interpersonal psychotherapy, Copyright (2000), reproduced with permission from American Psychological Association. No further reproduction or distribution is permitted.

Solution Focused	CBT	Psychodynamic
1. Identifying the client's preferred future, usually using the miracle question 2. The assumption that change is constant 3. Identification of times when the problem is less severe (search for exceptions) 4. Practitioner's assumption that the client has all the resources and skills necessary to enact their preferred future 5. The practitioner leads from "one step behind" 6. Use of complimentary language by the practitioner	1. Emphasizes homework and outside of session activities 2. Direction of session activity 3. Teaching skills to cope with symptoms 4. Focus on a patient's future experiences 5. Providing the patient with information about his or her treatment, disorder, or symptoms 6. Focuses on a patient's cognitive/intrapersonal experience (specifically illogical or irrational thoughts and beliefs)	1. Focus on affect and the expression of patients' emotion 2. Exploration of patients' attempts to avoid topics or engage in activities that hinder the progress of therapy 3. The identification of patterns in patients' actions, thoughts, feelings, experiences, and relationships 4. Emphasis on past experiences 5. Focus on patients' interpersonal experiences 6. Emphasis on the therapeutic relationship 7. Exploration of patients' wishes, dreams, or fantasies

unique based on how it was conceptualised in the literature. This identified six components that were described as essential and unique (as collated in Table 2.1).

Typical Cognitive Behavioural Therapy (CBT) and Psychodynamic approaches have similarly had their essential and unique components identified in previous research (Blagys & Hilsenroth, 2000; Blagys & Hilsenroth, 2002). We can compare Solution Focused approaches to CBT and Psychodynamic approaches in this way and begin to consider what is unique about being Solution Focused.

The use of homework and outside-of-session activities was deemed an essential and unique technique within CBT by Blagys and Hilsenroth (2002). Although this has been deemed an essential part of SFBT by many, it is not thought of as unique. In CBT and Psychodynamic approaches, we see an emphasis on either the patient's future or past experiences. Whilst in Solution Focused approaches, a client's present, past, and future are explored in the context of identifying their preferred future – noting exceptions to the problem or instances of the preferred future that have already happened – this approach could not be said to be unique to Solution Focused Practice.

Whilst CBT and Psychodynamic approaches place more emphasis on understanding the causation of the problem, how it is maintained, and coaching specific skills to cope with a particular presenting problem, Solution Focused approaches focus more on whatever seems to work for each unique client, *regardless* of the presenting problem.

Indeed, in Solution Focused Practice we do not even need to understand why something works, just that it brings about the desired change. Being Solution Focused seems to concentrate us much more on the assumption that change will happen – with the worker taking a stance that the client can and will achieve that change. In Solution Focused approaches, we also see the worker taking this 'one step behind' position, accepting that the client is the expert as well as the person to direct the session, with the worker skillfully supporting from behind without imposing an agenda. This seems to contrast with CBT, where the therapist directs the session's activity, or Psychodynamic approaches, where the therapist may specifically address things that they believe the client is trying to avoid.

Open Dialogue is another approach that has been designed for use in mental health crisis situations. This is a flexible, network-based approach to treatment which prioritises continuity and open discussion between the client and those in their network (Seikkula & Arnkil, 2006). Whilst both Open Dialogue and Solution Focused Practice stipulate that therapeutic work should be kept within the client's frame of reference and language, focused on what the client deems to be important (without imposing any particular agenda), there are some differences.

Open Dialogue describes an approach to facilitating discussions within a network, exploring how the client and those around them perceive the presenting problem, as well as the ways they believe things can move forward. Promoting dialogue is the main aim of the approach, with change coming second. Solution Focused Practice prioritises discussions which facilitate change rather than necessarily exploring the problem that brought the client to the practitioner (although, of course, space should be given to discussing the problem if the client wishes to discuss it). Open Dialogue also places great importance on continuity of care and responsibility within the client's network, whereas Solution Focused Practice provides a way of having discussions that can be used in any interaction, even if that is brief and limited to one encounter.

Solution Focused Practice appears to have now moved beyond specific required steps as described by de Shazer or Gingerich and Peterson and more towards an overall approach to conversations. McKergow (2016) has outlined this way of working and calls it 'SFBT 2.0'.

This model is primarily based on BRIEF's style of Solution Focused Practice (Iveson & McKergow, 2016; Shennan, 2019), which has been highly influential for the contributors to this book. Following on from the original conceptualisations of the approach, the model is characterised by some differences in how it is delivered.

1 More descriptive than action language, to immerse a client in their description rather than to seek interventions.
2 Questions are not just questions but open up 'rooms' of conversation that can be moved between.
3 The use of best hopes as themes for the work as opposed to setting goals which may or may not explicitly be met.
4 Preferred futures and scales are being used to enrich descriptions of desired change rather than to identify particular behaviours.
5 Asking about instances of preferred futures already happening rather than searching for exceptions to the problem.
6 No breaks, compliments, or interventions.
7 Ending without tasks or actions but with a summary demonstrating active listening.

McKergow does not advocate a move towards this new form of SFBT but rather reflects on a shift that has already occurred in practice. This Solution Focused Practice (as we call it in this book) – which can be used in a variety of settings, not just therapy – primarily centres on obtaining a client's best hopes for talking, using additional techniques to facilitate the description of a life containing best hopes, that can start to be lived the next day. This simplicity and adaptability have facilitated Solution Focused Practice's adoption well beyond therapy settings (Gingerich & Peterson, 2013; Neipp & Beyebach, 2024) and to the environments of mental health crises that we will be exploring.

What is it that makes Solution Focused Practice stand out? The Wampold (2015) contextual model of psychotherapy benefits suggests there are three pathways to positive outcomes in therapy: first, the therapeutic relationship; second, client expectations; and third, specific ingredients of a particular approach.

The therapeutic relationship has been investigated the most thoroughly in the literature, with numerous publications exploring the impact of different facets on therapy outcomes (Browne et al., 2021). Broadly speaking, modern psychotherapies conceptualise positive therapeutic relationships as those with positive interpersonal connections, supportive roles, and agreement between the therapist and client. In Solution Focused Practice, this is the core of the approach, where the worker views the client as the expert, leads from 'one step behind', and models the assumption that the client is skilled in their ability to achieve their desired future. With regards to expectations, clients are more likely to experience positive therapy outcomes if they believe the therapy will help and the more internal their locus of control (Browne et al., 2021). They are more likely to believe therapy can help if the therapist's explanations fit with their worldview (Wampold, 2015). Since Solution Focused Practice focuses on the client's best hopes, preferred future, and whatever they deem important (as opposed to imposing topics chosen by the therapist), it inherently promotes client expectations.

What are the specific ingredients of Solution Focused Practice which lead to its success? Being entirely based around whatever the client deems important allows the approach to be generic and adaptable, supporting the client in whatever they choose to work on rather than imposing a particular idea of 'healthy' or 'well'. The focus on the present and assuming change will happen – rather than focusing on unravelling the causation of a problem – is empowering and supports clients to make positive changes.

Similarly, the acceptance of the client's worldview, providing support towards their preferred future, and the practitioner's assumption they have the skills and resources to make these changes is also empowering and motivating (as opposed to highlighting deficits that need to be changed).

Asking questions about best hopes being lived out in the future, exploring this in detail using various techniques, and the power of someone hearing themselves say what it is that they want (and what this would look like) can make for real and lasting change. These factors, along with the experience of realising that problems are not always occurring, can provide the context for a shift away from a perception of overwhelming problems to one of being able to manage effectively and being able to move towards a future that will be better.

Solution Focused Practice is, therefore, particularly well suited to working with individuals in crisis. The definition of crisis that we use in this book is 'when you feel at breaking point, and you need urgent help' (MIND, 2020). The client's own frame of reference is crucial. By asking for details about the client's preferred future and exploring small steps towards it, appropriate and realistic ways to move forward from the crisis situation can be explored. Given that the original conceptualisations of SFBT were designed to be brief, delivered in however many sessions a client deems necessary – even if that is only one session (Henden, 2017) – this makes it suited to settings where intervention needs to be impactful in a short space of time.

As the work is to be shaped by the client's worldview, Solution Focused Practice provides a model that can be seen as cross-cultural and able to fit with perspectives and interpretations that may be outside of typical 'Western' models (Lee, 2003). The ability to understand the crisis from the individual's context and to support them in identifying viable solutions and outcomes based on their own values and socio-cultural background optimises the possibility for change. This is particularly important when we consider minoritised groups and the disproportionate number of individuals from non-White and non-Western backgrounds – particularly young Black males – who are detained under the Mental Health Act 1983 and diagnosed with severe mental illness (Gajwani et al., 2016). Ensuring we use models that seek to understand and empower individuals and can take into consideration their unique perspectives, values, and backgrounds is crucial, and Solution Focused Practice supports this.

There are some descriptions of Solution Focused approaches used specifically in crisis intervention: quite generally (Greene & Lee, 2015) and with adolescents (Hopson & Kim, 2004). These descriptions, while broadly following the typical approach discussed so far, highlight where the approach may require a slightly different focus.

Since Solution Focused approaches do not explore the problem in-depth, work can begin quickly to support the client in moving forward. However, more emphasis in crisis intervention may be given to allow the client to describe their current situation, should they wish to, to ensure they feel affirmed and heard (Greene & Lee, 2015; Hopson & Kim, 2004).

It may be particularly important to use the practitioner's judgement to gauge whether the client is ready to talk about change before moving to describe a preferred future (Greene & Lee, 2015), so as to avoid failing to acknowledge the seriousness of their situation. Techniques such as the use of relationship questions (what would others notice about you?) or rating scales can give multiple indicators of change (Greene & Lee, 2015; Hopson & Kim, 2004), which will be crucial to building vivid descriptions of the future that the client wants.

Identifying solution patterns used in the past and strengths the client has is particularly important for empowering clients in the current crisis situation (Greene & Lee, 2015), when it may be difficult to imagine a future without the problem (Hopson & Kim, 2004). Importantly, although specific assessments of safety or risk are not described as steps within the approach, these should be happening throughout the therapeutic work, and if immediate intervention to ensure a client's safety is required, this should not be proscribed. Evan George will refer to a 'twin-tracked' approach to statutory roles alongside therapeutic interventions later in the book.

Reviews of SFBT demonstrate a breadth of contexts that the approach is being delivered and researched in, as well as its effectiveness in a number of areas, including in mental health (Żak & Pękala, 2024; Vermeulen-Oskam et al., 2024). However, such reviews often highlight a lack of large, 'high quality' empirical studies that other therapeutic approaches, such as CBT, have developed. In particular, although descriptions of Solution Focused approaches to crisis intervention have been written about, there is very little published empirical research formally evidencing their use in this specific context. Current, ongoing, large-scale studies, such as the ASSURED and SASH studies that are described by Rose McCabe and colleagues in their chapter, will soon remedy this. From the accounts we find currently published in the literature, the results are promising. Rhodes and Jakes (2002) describe their findings from a case study using SFBT with an individual experiencing a psychotic crisis. Exploration of the client's desired future using

SFBT accepted the client's reality and what they wanted. This enabled the client to feel they could take control of their life and overcome their troubles. They reported the client was motivated and engaged and was able to identify concrete things they could do to change their situation.

Several research studies have explored the use of Solution Focused approaches with individuals reporting suicide risk (Jerome et al., 2024), including in inpatient settings, counselling, and tele-mental health. These studies found reduced suicide risk and a positive impact on a range of psychopathology-related outcomes (Ayar & Sabanciogullari, 2020; Baijesh & Suresh Kumar, 2018; Rhee et al., 2005).

Other research has explored the use of Solution Focused approaches, specifically in emergency department settings, with individuals presenting after self-harm or with suicide risk. These studies found positive perceptions and increased confidence in staff delivering the approach, as well as reduced re-presentations and a positive impact on other psychopathology and wellbeing related outcomes that were maintained over a follow-up period (Laydon et al., 2008; McAllister et al., 2009; Tapolaa et al., 2010; Wiseman, 2003). These studies provide some initial encouraging evidence of the use of Solution Focused Practice as an intervention in crisis situations. Whilst empirically, the evidence base is small, anecdotally, there is a wealth of encouraging reports of its use that just have not yet been formally demonstrated in the literature (Henden, 2017).

The remainder of this book provides accounts of Solution Focused Practice being used by professionals from a variety of backgrounds to demonstrate the impact of the approach on individuals in mental health crises. We hope that readers can identify with the scenarios and stories presented and see the difference that Solution Focused Practice can make.

References

Ayar, D., & Sabanciogullari, S. (2020). The effect of a solution-oriented approach in depressive patients on social functioning levels and suicide probability. *Perspectives in Psychiatric Care*, *57*(1). https://doi.org/10.1111/ppc.12554.

Baijesh, A., & Suresh Kumar, P. (2018). Solution Focused Brief Therapy (SFBT) In the treatment of depression and suicidal ideation: A case study. *Case Studies Journal ISSN (2305–509X)*, *7*(1), 61–65.

Blagys, M. D., & Hilsenroth, M. J. (2000). Distinctive features of short-term psychodynamic-interpersonal psychotherapy: A review of the comparative psychotherapy process literature. *Clinical Psychology: Science and Practice*, *7*(2), 167–188. https://doi.org/10.1093/clipsy.7.2.167.

Blagys, M. D., & Hilsenroth, M. J. (2002). Distinctive activities of cognitive-behavioral therapy. A review of the comparative psychotherapy process literature. *Clinical Psychology Review*, *22*(5), 671–706. https://doi.org/10.1016/s0272–7358(01)00117–9.

Browne, J., Cather, C., & Mueser, K. T. (2021). *Common factors in psychotherapy*. Oxford University Press. https://doi.org/10.1093/acrefore/9780190236557.013.79.

De Shazer, S., Berg, I., Lipchik, E., Nunnally, E., Molnar, A., Gingerich, W., & Weiner-Davis, M. (1986). Brief therapy: Focused solution development. *Family Process*, *25*(2), 207–221.

Gajwani, R., Parsons, H., Birchwood, M., & Singh, S. P. (2016). Ethnicity and detention: are Black and minority ethnic (BME) groups disproportionately detained under the

Mental Health Act 2007? *Soc Psychiatry Psychiatr Epidemiol, 51*(5), 703–711. https://doi.org/10.1007/s00127-016-1181-z.

Gingerich, W. J., & Peterson, L. T. (2013). Effectiveness of solution-focused brief therapy: A systematic qualitative review of controlled outcome studies. *Research on Social Work Practice, 23*(3), 266–283. https://doi.org/10.1177/1049731512470859.

Greene, G. J., & Lee, M.-Y. (2015). How to work with clients' strengths in crisis intervention: A solution-focused approach. In *Crisis intervention handbook: Assessment, treatment, and research* (4th ed., pp. 69–98). Oxford University Press.

Henden, J. (2017). *Preventing suicide: The solution focused approach*. John Wiley & Sons Ltd. https://doi.org/10.1002/9780470774120.

Hopson, L. M., & Kim, J. S. (2004). A solution-focused approach to crisis intervention with adolescents. *Journal of Evidence-Based Social Work, 1*(2–3), 93–110. https://doi.org/10.1300/J394v01n02_07.

Iveson, C., & McKergow, M. (2016). Brief therapy: Focused description development. *Journal of Solution Focused Practices, 2*(1).

Jerome, L., Masood, S., Henden, J., Bird, V., & Ougrin, D. (2024) Solution-focused approaches for treating self-injurious thoughts and behaviours: A scoping review. *BMC Psychiatry, 24*, 646. https://doi.org/10.1186/s12888-024-06101-7.

Jerome, L., McNamee, P., Abdel-Halim, N., Elliot, K., & Woods, J. (2023). Solution-focused approaches in adult mental health research: A conceptual literature review and narrative synthesis [Review]. *Frontiers in Psychiatry, 14*. https://doi.org/10.3389/fpsyt.2023.1068006.

Laydon, C., Mackenzie, S., Jones, S., & Wilson-Stonestreet, K. (2008). *Solution-focused therapy for clients who self-harm*. Nursing Times.

Lee, M. Y. (2003). A solution-focused approach to cross-cultural clinical social work practice utilizing cultural strengths. *Families in Society, 84*(3), 385–395. https://doi.org/10.1606/1044-3894.118.

McAllister, M., Moyle, W., Billett, S., & Zimmer-Gembeck, M. (2009). 'I can actually talk to them now': Qualitative results of an educational intervention for emergency nurses caring for clients who self-injure. *Journal of Clinical Nursing, 18*(20), 2838–2845. https://doi.org/10.1111/j.1365–2702.2008.02540.x.

McKergow, M. (2016). SFBT 2.0: The next generation of solution-focused brief therapy has already arrived. *Journal of Solution Focused Practices, 2*(2), Article 3.

Mental Health Act. (1983). *Mental Health Act 1983*. (legislation.gov.uk).

MIND. (2020). *Crisis services and planning*. Retrieved August 27, 2024, from www.mind.org.uk/information-support/guides-to-support-and-services/crisis-services/#:~:text=What's%20a%20mental%20health%20crisis,%2C%20or%20feeling%20very%20paranoid).

Neipp, M.-C., & Beyebach, M. (2024). The global outcomes of solution-focused brief therapy: A revision. *The American Journal of Family Therapy, 52*(1), 110–127. https://doi.org/10.1080/01926187.2022.2069175.

Rhee, W., Merbaum, M., Strube, M., & Self, S. (2005). Efficacy of brief telephone psychotherapy with callers to a suicide hotline. *Suicide and Life-Threatening Behavior, 35*(3), 317–328. https://doi.org/10.1521/suli.2005.35.3.317.

Rhodes, J., & Jakes, S. (2002). Using solution-focused therapy during a psychotic crisis: A case study. *Clinical Psychology & Psychotherapy, 9*(2), 139–148. https://doi.org/10.1002/cpp.329.

Seikkula, J., & Arnkil, T. E. (2006). *Dialogical meetings in social networks*. Karnac Books.

Shennan, G. (2019). *Solution-focused practice: Effective communication to facilitate change*. Bloomsbury Publishing. https://books.google.co.uk/books?id=OB5HEAAAQBAJ.

Tapolaa, V., Lappalainen, R., & Wahlstrom, J. (2010). Brief intervention for deliberate self harm: An exploratory study. *Suicidology Online, 1*, 95–108.

Vermeulen-Oskam, E., Franklin, C., van't Hof, L. P. M., Stams, G. J. J. M., van Vugt, E. S., Assink, M., Veltman, E. J., Froerer, A. S., Staaks, J. P. C., & Zhang, A. (2024). The current evidence of solution-focused brief therapy: A meta-analysis of psychosocial outcomes and moderating factors. *Clinical Psychology Review, 114*, 102512. https://doi.org/10.1016/j.cpr.2024.102512.

Waltz, J., Addis, M. E., Koerner, K., & Jacobson, N. S. (1993). Testing the integrity of a psychotherapy protocol: Assessment of adherence and competence. *Journal of Consulting and Clinical Psychology, 61*(4), 620–630. https://doi.org/10.1037/0022–006X.61.4.620.

Wampold, B. E. (2015). How important are the common factors in psychotherapy? An update. *World Psychiatry, 14*(3), 270–277. https://doi.org/10.1002/wps.20238.

Watzlawick, P., Weakland, J. H., & Fisch, R. (1974). *Change: Principles of problem formation and problem resolution.* W. W. Norton.

Wiseman, S. (2003). Brief intervention: Reducing the repetition of deliberate self-harm. *Nursing Times, 99*(35), 34–36.

Żak, A. M., & Pękala, K. (2024). Effectiveness of solution-focused brief therapy: An umbrella review of systematic reviews and meta-analyses. *Psychotherapy Research*, 1–13. https://doi.org/10.1080/10503307.2024.2406540.

Chapter 3

The impact of Solution Focused conversations on the structure of the brain (and why we should all be using this approach to treat trauma)

Adam S. Froerer

Traumatic events and incidents are happening around the globe on a daily basis. The media airs these trauma-filled stories and rebroadcasts the negative impacts of these events throughout the 24-hour news cycle. Individuals and groups in marginalized situations are particularly at risk and experience a compounding effect due to oppression, but no one is spared the impacts of experiencing or witnessing one or more traumatic events at some point in their lifetime (Briere & Scott, 2015). Trauma has become a ubiquitous human experience. Many are suffering, and trauma is contributing to the mental health crisis we are seeing worldwide (Hogan & Goldman, 2020). However, since trauma has not completely crippled society, and since we can still see growth, development, success, triumphs, happiness, love, and healing, there is still hope. This chapter will outline how Solution Focused language has the power to shift trauma to resilience, and (through inclusive support) shift mental health crises towards safety and hope.

The physical and psychological impacts of trauma

According to the American Psychological Association (2024),

> Trauma is an emotional response to a terrible event like an accident, crime, natural disaster, physical or emotional abuse, neglect, experiencing or witnessing violence, death of a loved one, war, and more. Immediately after the event, shock and denial are typical. Longer term reactions include unpredictable emotions, flashbacks, strained relationships, and even physical symptoms like headaches or nausea.
>
> (www.apa.org/topics/trauma)

Two-thirds of the general population will endure at least one traumatic experience at some point in their lives, and one in five will encounter a traumatic experience in any given year (Galea et al., 2005). It is clear from research that individuals seeking clinical mental help are at increased risk of having experienced childhood and/or adulthood trauma (Kessler et al., 2010; Van der Kolk, 2003). The overall wellbeing

DOI: 10.4324/9781003519225-3

of individuals who have experienced childhood trauma decreases significantly with an increased likelihood of poor mental health, severe physical health problems, and premature death (Sweeney et al., 2016; Wallace, 2024). This epidemic of trauma is one contributing factor to the mental health crisis that is growing in many places throughout the world.

Traditional approaches to treating trauma and Post-Traumatic Stress Disorder

Given the significant prevalence of trauma and the resulting post-traumatic stress disorder (PTSD), it is important for us to understand what works to help people manage and overcome PTSD and trauma symptoms. Trauma-focused approaches are the foremost recommended treatments for clients experiencing PTSD, despite the fact that between one-third and one-half of clients who receive this treatment 'do not optimally respond to these treatments' (p. 768) and continue to display persistent PTSD symptoms even after treatment (Keyan et al., 2024).

Trauma-focused (T-F) refers to a range of treatments (i.e., CBT, EMDR, and exposure therapy) that all share similar components. Clients referred to T-F treatments are usually required to 1) revisit memories of the trauma; 2) process the associated emotions of revisiting the trauma; and 3) typically try to alter the negative thoughts about the trauma or self with some type of cognitive restructuring (Keyan et al., 2024). Given the heavy focus on re-experiencing the trauma, the associated negative emotions, and being viewed as a person with negative (and faulty) perceptions and self-images, it is no wonder that many clients do not improve as a result of this treatment. In fact, some clinicians have even argued that this T-F approach causes increased attrition from therapy, is unethical, and can even retraumatize clients (Jones, 2018). It is vital that we provide clients managing trauma a better option to treatment that does not cause them harm or contribute to the mental health crisis we are experiencing.

Wellbeing

We choose to believe that accompanying every trauma experience is a companion experience of resilience, strength, and the ability to overcome. Anyone who has survived a trauma for the next hour, the next day, the next year, or over much of their post-trauma lifetime has demonstrated resilience, demonstrated a desire for increased wellbeing, and demonstrated hope for possible change and improvement. The simple fact that they have not given up, have not passed away, and have not allowed the trauma to completely consume their every thought means that they have built resilience and increased capacity to cope. Clinicians should feel duty-bound to highlight this resilience, build on this strength, and aid healing with an approach that does not increase the likelihood of harm. Solution Focused Brief Therapy (SFBT) is such an approach.[1]

The neurochemistry of trauma and Solution-Focused Brief Therapy

Extensive research has been conducted to evaluate the neurochemical and physiological factors and impacts of trauma on the human brain (Sherin & Nemeroff, 2022). It should be made very clear that many factors (genetic, gender, early developmental, and physical factors) impact the effects of trauma, and it cannot be definitively stated what the impact will be for any given individual. However, some general trends are worth considering. Sherin and Nemeroff (2022) indicate that at least three brain structures correlate with the presence of post-traumatic stress disorder (PTSD) in trauma sufferers: the hippocampus, the amygdala, and the medial prefrontal cortex. The hippocampus, which controls the stress response, declarative memory, and the contextual aspects of fear-conditioning, is reduced in overall volume in individuals managing PTSD. This smaller hippocampus results in hyper-fear response, lower stress management, and ambiguity within memories. Beyond the hippocampus, the amygdala is also impacted within those managing PTSD. The amygdala regulates emotional and stress responses and regulates emotional learning. When managing a trauma, the amygdala increases activity and sends messages to other parts of the brain, indicating learning should slow or suspend and that all efforts should be made to manage the increased presence of stress. Therefore, emotional decision-making takes over, and logical decision-making is negatively impacted. Finally, the medial prefrontal cortex (PFC) also decreases in overall volume. This smaller PFC inhibits control over stress response and emotional activity, further letting the emotional trauma response flow unfettered. As a result of this, in order to help individuals manage trauma better, the treatment should work to counter the impact on these brain structures.

SFBT is a useful treatment that could have a positive impact on these brain structures and systems.

Keyan et al. (2024) recommend that effective therapy approaches should include each of the following elements in order to help reverse the physiological impacts of trauma. Effective therapy should 1) focus on improving emotion; 2) remove rumination of negative thought patterns; 3) decrease dysphoria; 4) improve executive functioning; 5) improve prosocial interactions; 6) address shame and guilt; and 7) let people choose their own form of treatment. SFBT is uniquely qualified and meets each of these recommendations. Kim and Franklin (2015) explain that SFBT increases positive emotions and leads the client to have a wider vision of future possibilities. This increased hope and optimism replaces negative thoughts and decreases dysphoria and depression. Through meaningful questions, clients are asked to describe in great detail the impact hope and healing will have on their meaningful loved ones, thus improving prosocial interactions. Clients also have the opportunity to focus on, and grow toward, their desired outcome (something that will be discussed later in the chapter), which changes their perception from guilt and shame to one of possibility and ability. Finally, SFBT honors clients' agency and autonomy from the beginning of the session – with the best hopes question – all the way to the end by allowing the client to determine when successful therapy should be concluded. SFBT is a superb alternative to traditional trauma-focused approaches. We should turn to SFBT to help treat the trauma-related crisis that is happening worldwide.

SFBT Diamond

Solution Focused Brief Therapy is a change-oriented and difference-oriented approach that aims to help clients achieve change through meaningful conversations. The Diamond Approach is a recent innovation to how Solution Focused Brief Therapy is conceptualized and carried out. The Diamond Approach was developed by Elliott Connie and Adam Froerer (2023). It is essentially 'a flowchart that comprises the five skills you need to master to do solution focused brief therapy effectively' (Connie & Froerer, 2023, pp. 95). These five skills: 1) obtaining a desired outcome; 2) having a history of the outcome descriptive conversation; 3) having resources for the outcome descriptive conversation; 4) having a future of the

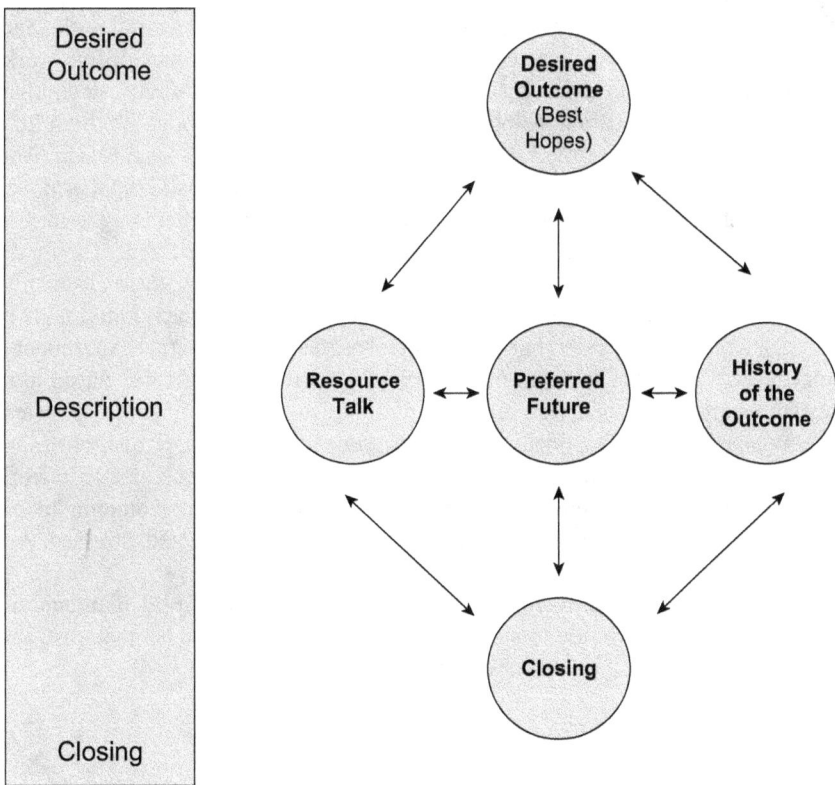

Figure 3.1 The Solution Focused Diamond, developed by Elliott Connie and Adam Froerer (2023).

outcome descriptive conversation; and 5) closing the session in a way that honors the client's agency and autonomy, have the power to change individual lives, alter the impact to trauma, and change the trajectory of the mental health crisis we are collectively experiencing.

The bulk of the rest of the chapter will use an anonymised case example, with additional commentary, to illustrate how SFBT can be effective at aiding a client in managing trauma in meaningful ways.

Case example background

Susan is a 55-year-old African-American woman. Susan married her husband at the age of 25 and quickly thereafter gave birth to a daughter named Martha. Susan endured emotional and psychological violence throughout her relationship with her husband. He regularly commented about Susan's weight, called her fat and ugly, commented that she wasn't pulling her fair share of the financial burden, and regularly commented that she was parenting 'all wrong', that she was 'going to ruin Martha', and that she wouldn't amount to anything. After seven years of enduring this trauma, Susan divorced her husband and moved out with Martha. Susan got a job working with special needs children. As part of this work, Susan was required to assist the children physically so they could accomplish day-to-day tasks like eating, using the restroom, and moving about the room. In a moment of panic, one of the large male students jumped away from Susan, who was unprepared for the sudden motion. This action caused Susan's right arm, her dominant arm, to be dislocated, and several tendons and ligaments were torn in the process. This injury resulted in the need for an emergency surgery. The injury and her ongoing interactions with the medical field further traumatized Susan. She had grown up with messages from her family of origin that Black individuals in America wouldn't be treated fairly by medical professionals and that experimental procedures were often inflicted on unsuspecting African Americans. Susan mistrusted her physician and was reluctant to complete the recommended physical therapy post-surgery. The doctor verbally reprimanded Susan and mentioned that if she didn't heal well, 'it will be your own fault'. Susan has been unable to work for the last six months, and her employer is threatening not to pay ongoing medical leave for much longer. Susan presents for therapy traumatized, stressed, and worried about the future.

The following will outline each of the components of an SFBT diamond approach session, will provide session dialogue between Susan and her therapist, and will be supplemented with author commentary.

Desired outcome

The first task within an SFBT session is to help the client articulate what they would like to get out of therapy, i.e., their desired outcome. A workable desired outcome is often a component of the client's identity they would like to change and see more of. The desired outcome is positive and may or may not have much to do with the presenting problem the client brings to therapy.

Therapist: Hi Susan. It is really nice to meet you. What are your best hopes for our work together?

Susan: I'm not really that hopeful. In fact, I'm pretty nervous and scared. I was injured at work, and I don't seem to be getting much better. I'm really scared that I'm going to get fired. I have been unable to attend work for the past six months.

Therapist: Wow, I can see why it might be hard to find hope in this moment. However, I'm wondering if you and I were somehow able to work through this fear and stress, if we were able to accomplish something really helpful, what would you most like to have happen as a result of our work together?

Susan: I guess I would like to feel better. I would like to be able to get back to work and be able to take care of my daughter well.

Therapist: That's amazing! If you were able to start to feel better, get back to work, and take care of your daughter like you would like to, what difference would that make to you?

Susan: If I could do that, I would feel like my old self again. I would be able to finally relax.

Therapist: And if you got to be your old self again and you were able to relax in just the right way, what impact would that have on you?

Susan: I would know that I was actually becoming who I am supposed to be. I would know that these setbacks wouldn't define me.

This exchange, although short, is really meaningful! Notice the therapist listens closely to Susan and regularly uses the exact language Susan uses. However, the therapist uses this language in a way that helps Susan articulate what she wants rather than asking her for further details about the trauma or the impact of the trauma. This immediately shifts Susan's thinking to what she would like and begins the process of reducing shame and guilt, broadening her perspective of options while reducing negative cognitions and improving her perspective about prosocial interactions. Each of these things is consistent with the effective therapy components outlined previously. In addition, Susan is in complete control of what the outcome will be and contributes significantly to the type of treatment she will receive. None of these questions further traumatize her or focus her attention on triggers or trauma flashbacks.

History of the outcome

A common misconception about SFBT is that it is an approach that only focuses on the future and may overlook or minimize the past. This is inaccurate. A hallmark of the Diamond Approach is that if someone can tell you what their desired outcome is, they must have experienced it previously! This means they have a history that is consistent with this desired outcome. When clients are asked to review their past, not so much for the trauma-related details, but for the desired outcome details, they get reacquainted with the best version of themselves, and they realize that they have separate histories (trauma history and desired outcome history) that have been living side by side the whole time.

Potentially, the trauma-related history has been taking up more space, or they have focused on it more, but through SFBT (and SFP) conversations, clients can realize that strength, resources, and resilience are all present in their desired outcome history and in their coping with trauma history. History of the outcome conversations allows the client to acknowledge their ability to survive despite the presence of trauma: they get to acknowledge that the version of themselves that they hope for is already within, and they get to reclaim this person.

Therapist: Susan, as you think back on your life, when have you been able to relax in a way that lets you know that you were your old self and that you were living up to the person you were supposed to be?

Susan: Man, that was a really long time ago, probably before I married my ex-husband. I didn't really get to be myself when I was with him.

Therapist: So it was before you got married. When would you say you were most able to be your old self and really relax?

Susan: I guess I would have to say back when I was in college. Even though I had a lot going on, and it was really stressful at times, I just felt like anything was possible. I just felt like I could accomplish anything I put my mind to. I haven't felt like that for a really long time.

Therapist: What was something that you noticed then that really told you, 'this is the real me'?

Susan: I loved to learn. I would sit in class and just soak things up. It was like there was nothing else in the world going on.

Therapist: Who knew you the best at that time that would have also picked up on the fact that you were relaxed in your learning and that you were preparing to be your real self?

Susan: Probably my roommate. She used to always tell me I was crazy because I was studying so much. But I just loved it.

This exchange is just one possible exchange about history that could have happened. You should notice that each of the therapist's utterances is formulated by incorporating Susan's language from her previous utterance. This pattern should be present throughout the entire session. In addition, notice that Susan mentioned her ex-husband (a source of her trauma) and that she mentioned that she hasn't felt her desired outcome for a long time. Both of these 'trauma pitfalls' were avoided by the therapist by using the language of the desired outcome to get a rich description of what was different about Susan at that time. By helping Susan remember that her true and relaxed self was present, the therapist is helping her remember what was different about her when she was living this way. Even though trauma isn't being overtly addressed (since the previously cited research mentions that this might actually do more harm), Susan is getting reacquainted with a version of herself that she would like to be. There is a parallel history that can be utilized in therapy to help Susan begin to view herself differently.

Resources for the outcome

One of the hallmarks of SFBT and SFP is the focus on strengths and resources. Nowhere is that more prevalent than in a Resources for the Outcome conversation. Clients are asked to acknowledge the skills, qualities, traits, or resources they possess that could contribute to the presence of the desired outcome. This is a conversation that puts a spotlight on the fact that, despite their trauma(s), the client has qualities that are beneficial and that can help in a variety of ways. This is also an opportunity for clients to realize that they are using resources each minute or each day to cope with and manage the impacts and symptoms of trauma. Resource conversations ask the client to acknowledge that even though the trauma is challenging to manage, they can manage it and heal.

Therapist: Susan, what do you already know about yourself that lets you know you're the kind of person who is capable of relaxing and getting back to your old self?

Susan: I'm not actually sure. I haven't felt like that since before my accident and my failed marriage.

Therapist: Think back to when you were in college; what skill did you use to relax and be your true self?

Susan: I guess I was organized and structured.

Therapist: What difference did it make to be organized and structured?

Susan: It helped me to be able to think ahead and plan for what was coming.

Therapist: When you plan and think ahead, what difference does it make for you in uncertain times?

Susan: It helps me to feel settled and to know that I can handle what's coming.

Therapist: What makes you good at handling things that are coming when you feel settled?

Susan: I think I just feel more confident.

You can notice that through this series of questions, the therapist helped Susan articulate skills like being organized and structured, being a planner, being someone who thinks ahead, and being someone who is settled and able to handle things. While Susan articulates these previously utilized skills, she is really building up a picture of the version of herself that is capable of dealing with trauma or anything else that comes her way. Even without directly addressing the trauma, Susan is refamiliarizing herself with the version of herself that can manage trauma the best.

Future of the outcome

Probably the most well-known component of SFBT is the emphasis on the future. Envisioning a future that is consistent with the desired outcome can help people realize that their best hopes are achievable. Previously, this kind of conversation was started with the 'miracle question' (de Shazer et al., 2007); however, in the Diamond Approach, using this specific question isn't necessary.

Therapist: Suppose tomorrow there is a shift or change that happens, and the relaxed, old, true version of you shows up. When would you be most likely to realize this change had happened?

Susan: I guess I would notice if my boss tried to call me.

Therapist: What would be the first thing you noticed that would let you know your old self was back, even if a stressful thing like your boss calling happened?

Susan: I would know that I could speak calmly and discuss the progress of my situation. I would think clearly and tell him what I needed.

Therapist: Would this be a different way for you to interact with him?

Susan: Yeah! Really different.

This sort of conversation would continue with the therapist asking about the smallest differences and details that would appear when Susan's old self was present. This 'walk through' of a day would bring to mind many things that would be impacted by the desired outcome. This walk-through would be experienced by Susan's brain, like events that were actually happening, not just events that she was talking about. This walk-through, like the other Diamond approach descriptions, would directly change Susan's amygdala with happy emotions, her hippocampus with a reorientation to past, present, and future, and her prefrontal cortex with logical thinking and decision-making that is based on her true self. Real change would be built one question and utterance at a time, using the client's own words and their own priorities.

Conclusion

SFBT is an excellent alternative to T-F approaches to trauma. It is a caring, compassionate approach that asks the client to reacquaint themselves with the very best of themselves. SFBT allows all people, especially marginalized individuals, to be taken seriously. They aren't asked to accommodate the dominant position or perspective. Their language is not only valued but used word for word by the clinician to develop meaning that is pertinent to their worldview and perspective. All individuals get to show up as themselves, feel valued, and work towards their own desired outcome. This 'best-self version' is more than capable of managing trauma symptoms in adaptive ways. This best-self version is full of hope! This best-self version is who the client really is!

Note

1 I refer to SFBT in this chapter because the context for my contribution is therapy. I am aware that other contributors to this book are using the term Solution Focused Practice (SFP) because this best describes their use of Solution Focused questions within their own workplace and professional role.

References

American Psychological Association. (2024). Retrieved September 19, 2024, from www. apa.org/topics/trauma.

Briere, J. N., & Scott, C. (2015). *Principles of trauma focused therapy: A guide to symptoms, evaluation, and treatment* (2nd ed.). Sage.

Connie, E. E., & Froerer, A. S. (2023). *The solution focused brief therapy diamond: A new approach to SFBT that will empower both practitioner and client to achieve the best outcomes*. Hay House Inc.

De Shazer, S., Dolan, Y., Korman, H., Trepper, T., McCollum, E., Berg, I. K. (2007). *More than Miracles: The state of the art of solution-focused brief therapy*. Routledge.

Galea, G., Nandi, A., & Vlahov, D. (2005). The epidemiology of post-traumatic stress disorder after disasters. *Epidemiologic Reviews, 27*, 78–91. https://doi.org/10.1093/epirev/mxi003.

Hogan, M. F., & Goldman, M. L. (2020). New opportunities to improve mental health crisis systems. *Psychiatric Services, 72*(2). https://doi.org/10.1176/appi.ps.202000114.

Jones, M. (2018). *The use of exposure therapy for patients with PTSD or a history of trauma* (Master's thesis, Pacific University). Retrieved from https://commons.pacificu.edu/spp/1417.

Kessler, R. C., McLaughlin, K. A., Green, J. G., Gruber, M. J., Sampson, N. A., Zaslavsky, A. M., & Williams, D. R. (2010). Childhood adversities and adult psychopathology in the WHO World Mental Health Surveys. *The British Journal of Psychiatry, 197*(5), 378–385. https://doi.org/10.1192/bjp.bp.110.080499.

Keyan, D., Garland, N., Choi-Christou, J., Tran, J., O'Donnell, M., & Bryant, R. A. (2024). A systematic review and meta-analysis of predictors of response to trauma-focused psychotherapy for posttraumatic stress disorder. *Psychological Bulletin, 150*(7), 767–797. https://doi.org/10.1037/bul0000438.

Kim, J. S., & Franklin, C. (2015). Understanding emotional change in solution-focused brief therapy: Facilitating positive emotions. *Best Practices in Mental Health, 11*(1), 25–41.

Sherin, J. E., & Nemeroff, C. B. (2022). Post-traumatic stress disorder: The neurobiological impact of psychological trauma. *Dialogues in Clinical Neuroscience, 13*(3), 263–278. https://doi.org/10.31887/DCNS.2011.13.2/jsherin.

Sweeney, A., Clement, S., Filson, B., & Kennedy, A. (2016). Trauma-informed mental healthcare in the UK: What is it and how can we further its development? *Mental Health Review Journal, 21*(3), 174–192. http://doi.org/10.1108/MHRJ-01-2015-0006.

Van der Kolk, B. A. (2003). The neurobiology of childhood trauma and abuse. *Child and Adolescent Psychiatric Clinics, 12*(2), 293–317. https://doi.org/10.1016/S1056–4993(03)00003–8.

Wallace, E. (2024). Different types of trauma affecting quality of life and mental well-being. *Journal of Psychological Research and Investigation*. https://doi.org/10.13140/RG.2.2.15979.76327.

Chapter 4

Extemporising Solution Focused Practice – using the approach moment by moment

Guy Shennan

Introduction

"Yes", I responded, after the editor of this book asked, "Would you like to write a chapter on unplanned uses of the Solution Focused approach?" That one-word answer – that "enormous yes", as the poet Philip Larkin (1990) called it – set in motion a process, a gathering momentum, which led to the words you are now reading arriving on the page.

So, one question can have a large impact, especially perhaps when the answer fits with or creates a direction that the respondent wants to go in. This chapter will explore how bits of Solution Focused Practice (SFP) can be used in everyday conversations, away from the therapy room, often on the spur of the moment. Such use is aided when the practitioner is ready with questions that connect with concerns they are hearing while simultaneously creating a possibility of forward movement. Beginning with a question that can be answered with the word "yes" is often a good start. Ready to read more?

Having completed my first course in Solution-Focused Brief Therapy (SFBT), I realised that my next task in becoming able to use the approach was to figure out how to apply it in my work role, given that I wasn't a therapist but a social worker working with children and families in a Social Services duty team. I was aided in this by my discovery that there are two ways of using SFP. One is as "a fully structured approach, in planned sessions", while the second is to use elements of it "in more opportunistic ways within the unplanned conversational contexts in which many helping professionals frequently find themselves" (Shennan, 2019, p. x). I found I could use it in both ways. At times, we arranged meetings in which we were able to follow the full Solution Focused (SF) structure (see Shennan, 2019, pp. 190–191, for an account of creating an optimal context for this), while I was also able to draw on aspects of the SF approach on many other occasions, including in the less planned parts of my job.

This chapter is about the second of these two ways. I will first suggest that certain features of SFP make it useable in this way and that a particular characterisation of SF work can help us see why this is the case. I will then set out some ideas that assist my readiness to respond in an SF way when an opportunity arises and give examples of such responses based on my own practice.

DOI: 10.4324/9781003519225-4

Solution Focused Practice and everyday conversations

What is it about SFP that lends itself to being both useable and potentially useful in everyday conversations, including brief and sometimes one-off encounters? We might note the original (and still current in therapy contexts) name of Solution-Focused *Brief* Therapy. In planned contexts, "brief" has become briefer over time, from up to 10 sessions in the Brief Therapy that preceded the SF variety (Weakland et al., 1974), decreasing to an average of five for the original SF team (de Shazer et al., 1986), and a later study at BRIEF in the UK showing an average of less than two sessions (Shennan & Iveson, 2011).

Among the reasons for this decrease is one that I believe sheds some light on why SFP can be used outside these planned contexts. An important early SF study (Gingerich et al., 1988) explored what therapists did that elicited "change talk" during sessions, that is, talk about positive (in the sense of desired by the client) change that has either already happened or might in the future. The study's findings encouraged the team to ask clients about such change ever earlier, and correspondingly *not to* ask about the problem, thus shortening the work as well as contributing to the development of SFP as we know it today.

In my view, just as important as these shifts in practice, for this chapter's purposes, was the focus on *change talk* by the client. SFP is usually defined by what the practitioner does, the types of questions asked, and the structures into which these questions are organised. Another way to characterise SF conversations is by *the type of talk that the client engages in during them*, or at least that which the practitioner aims to encourage and elicit.

Whereas Gingerich and his colleagues use the all-embracing term *change talk* to refer to this, I suggest this can usefully be separated into *future talk* and *progress talk*. We can then say that a practitioner is using an SF approach in a conversation if they invite future talk – about what the person hopes for; what they want instead of a problem; what "better" might look like; what difference this might make; or a combination of these – and/or progress talk – about exceptions to problems; any times when things are even a little bit better, or have been better previously; about any movement in a desired direction; about how they are keeping going; or a combination of these.

We can also add that the practitioner can do this however that conversation arises, in whatever context, and for however long it lasts, whether for less than a minute or more than an hour. This is because SFP is not a programmatic approach, where a therapeutic procedure has to be followed and completed, and there is also no requirement for the "client" to return for a follow-up session. Any amount of future talk or progress talk, or a mixture of both, could be helpful, and opportunities to invite people to think and talk in such ways frequently arise. Let me provide you with one now, by way of an example. I don't imagine you were planning to use SFP while reading this chapter. However, what if I told you I was stuck and did not know what to write next? How might you draw on aspects of SFP in order to offer some help?

You could invite me into some future talk by asking one or more questions like these (and just one on its own might be useful, as I have often found with a supervisor who is able to ask me SF questions):

What would you like to be instead of stuck?
Suppose when you next return to your desk to have another go, you find you are no longer stuck. What's the first thing you'd notice about yourself?
And the next thing? . . .

Or you could try some questions to encourage some progress talk, including progress in the past:

How have you managed to write what you have so far?
When you've felt stuck previously, what have you found helpful?

Rather than following a programme, the SF practitioner follows the answers of the client and uses the client's words and language to formulate their successive questions. This is what is meant by saying that SFP is a conversational approach, and this also helps aspects of the SF approach to be used in everyday conversations. Furthermore, the attention that SF practitioner gives to the words and language of the client – and to their actual words rather than a paraphrase of them – can have an equalising effect. Using the client's own language is especially important for people who experience structural oppression, which an imposition of professional language can add to. Staying with the client's words can help to ensure that the client's hopes, preferences, and meanings are privileged.

Useful ideas

There are a number of ideas and assumptions it is useful to carry around with you, which can help you spot opportunities to use some SFP. One involves always being ready to hear the phrase *at the moment* when someone tells you about a problem they have. Even when this isn't said out loud, it can usually be assumed. This idea was actually at work in the questions listed in the previous section that you might have asked me if I had told you I was feeling stuck writing this chapter. Drawing on the work of O'Hanlon and Beadle (1996), you could have prefaced these questions by acknowledging my problem but then lacing this acknowledgement with this possibility-laden phrase: "So you're feeling stuck *at the moment?*". That this is unlikely to be the case forever creates the possibility of future talk. That it can't have always been the case (otherwise, no writing would have been done so far) means that progress talk must be possible.

A second idea, related to the first, is that *nothing happens all the time*, not even difficult problems. It can feel like they do, and people talk *as if* they do – "We are always fighting"; "I feel terrible all the time"; "I can't do anything about it" – but this is unlikely to be the actual case. Once again, a useful initial response arising from this idea is to acknowledge the problem while adding possibility by reducing the *always* to *sometimes* – "So you're feeling bad *a lot of the time,* at the moment".

This idea was central in the initial development of SFP as the original team in Milwaukee realised that there must always be *exceptions* to the problem (de Shazer et al., 1986): times when it might have happened but didn't, or happens with less intensity, or for a shorter period. Coming across this idea as a social worker, I realised there would be ample opportunity to act on it, as everyone I was working with had problems and told me about them. The first time I did so was with a family consisting of a single mum and her two sons – aged 14 and 12 – who were always fighting, or so it seemed.

Hearing about one of these fights, triggered by the younger boy using something belonging to his older brother without asking, I enquired whether there had been a time when that had happened, and they had resolved it without fighting. It turned out there had been, though, at that stage of my SF career, I wasn't as ready to take advantage of this opportunity as I came to be later when I became familiar with the types of SF questions useful in these moments. On hearing an exception of this type, it is almost always possible to follow up along these lines:

What happened instead of the problem (in this case, the fight)?
What did you do?
How did you do that?
Was that a good way of doing it? What difference did it make?
When else have you managed to resolve things in that better sort of way?

A third idea, also related, is that as well as having difficulties, there will be things happening in the person's life *that they want to be happening* and that they want to continue to happen. The importance of this idea to the original development of SFP cannot be overstated, as can be seen in the recent English translation of a book chapter published originally in French (Hopwood & de Shazer, 2021, available online). A family listed a large number of problems, all in vague terms, and unsure of how to proceed, the therapy team decided to do something different and asked the family to list all the things they noticed that they *didn't want to change* and report back at the next session. In addition to their list of what they didn't want to change, the family reported positive changes related to the problems they had come with. This led to an increasing focus by the Milwaukee team on positive aspects of people's lives that they wanted to continue.

Keeping this idea in mind can be useful in a number of ways, such as in situations where someone is stuck in problem talk. One way begins – after sufficient acknowledgement of how difficult the problems are – by inviting in that useful word, "Yes", by asking, "Can I ask you something a bit different?" The answer "Yes" can be followed by saying that many people in difficult situations like this find it useful to consider what is happening in their life that they want to continue, even though this can involve some hard thinking. Such comments can help a shift away from problem talk towards talking about things that are wanted, legitimising this different type of talking, and supporting the person to do the thinking required for it.

If it is hard to talk about these things at such a moment, a second way to use this idea is to give the person questions to take away with them. Luc Isebaert (2017, p. 99), an SF psychiatrist from Belgium, described his "Three Questions for a Good Life" as a way of orienting the client to a more satisfactory present:

What did I do that I am happy with?
What did someone else do that I am happy with, or that I am grateful for?
What do I see around me, what do I hear, feel, smell, taste that I am happy with or grateful for?

His team printed these questions on business cards and fridge magnets and encouraged their clients to look at and try to answer them each day. Isebaert (2017, p. 101) reported that these questions improved the quality of life of their "chronic clients", who had either alcohol, somatic, or psychological problems.

A fourth potentially useful idea is one I have called *the* SF assumption (Shennan, 2019, pp. 30–31). Related to the planned context, this can be stated: if someone has come for help, then they must be hoping that something will come from that. However, it can be assumed more generally that if someone is talking to another person who is in a helping role, then they must have some hope from that talking. The opening question of a planned piece of SF work is frequently: "What are your best hopes from our work together?" or some variant thereof. Reworded slightly to fit the context, this question can be potentially used in any situation where a person is choosing to talk with someone in a helping role. For example, I found it extremely useful while taking telephone calls in a duty social work team, especially when a call had been going on for some time, and I had begun to feel a little lost in the midst of hearing about a complicated situation. I could then say: "Can I just check, when you decided to make this call, what were you hoping might happen as a result of it?" This helped to extricate us from the thickets we had been caught up in, setting us on a clearer way forward. Similarly, David Unwin reports that using this question in his consultations as a GP tended to strip away the long histories that some patients launched into, which there was neither the time for nor were relevant usually to what was to be done. He found that it was "more efficient if the conversation is experienced in the context of (the patient's) 'best hopes'" (Unwin, 2005, p. 12).

Listening with a constructive ear

What we listen for, and therefore hear, will also add to our ability to respond in SF ways. To listen with a constructive ear, a phrase associated with Eve Lipchik of the original Milwaukee team (Shennan, 2019, p. 18), leads us to hear snippets of future talk, or progress talk, in the midst of whatever else is being said.

Suppose someone reports a difficult situation they are in as follows:

I'm fed up at the moment, feeling very down. It's getting cold, and I can't afford to put the heating on. It's hard to get out of bed in the morning; last weekend, especially, was a nightmare. I've hardly been out and not really spoken to anyone.

Before reading on, take a moment to think about any snippets you see there, explicit or implicit, of progress or future talk.

A "both/and" perspective, similar to the acknowledgement *and* possibility we saw previously, is useful. Listening with a constructive ear does not mean closing our ears to difficulties, but hearing *both* the problem *and* other aspects of a situation that can lead to the development of future and progress talk. For example, this person both found it hard to get out of bed and managed to, an observation that can lead to a response such as, "So it was hard to get out of bed – how did you do it?". A constructive ear also hears *differences*: one being signalled by the word "especially". As the "weekend, especially, was a nightmare", it might be worth asking, "What was different in the week that made it not as difficult?".

Certain other words used also point to exceptions, like "hardly", which suggests that the person went out on at least one occasion. "How come? How did you do that? What difference did that make?". The phrase "not really" might suggest similar questions. Finally, notice those three words again – "at the moment" – after the statement of being fed up. They open the door, even if just a crack, to talk of a different, more desired future. Questions like these might push it open a little further:

How would you like to be feeling instead?
Suppose you weren't feeling quite so fed up; what would be different?
What would be the first small sign that you are feeling a little better?
Who else would notice? What would they notice about you?

Starting with a Yes

A well-known book on negotiating is called *Getting to Yes* (Fisher et al., 2011), though another way to open the door to an SF conversation is to *start* with a yes, as noted at the beginning of this chapter. We will finish with a couple of examples of doing this, which might provide a hint of why James Joyce called yes "the most positive word in the human language" (Ellmann, 1982, p. 522).

Constructive ears also listen out for what someone wants, which is sometimes quite straightforward to hear, as when I was introduced to someone as their new social worker, and their first words to me were, "I don't want a social worker; I just want to live a normal life!" As always, acknowledging what they did not want was essential and paved the way for asking, "Would you be willing to work with me towards the sort of normal life that you want and that would satisfy my department that we don't have to be in your life?". After they answered, "Yes", I was able to invite both future talk – "Suppose you woke up tomorrow to the sort of life that's right for you and that would get us off your back, what would you notice? Can you describe some of it?" – and progress talk – "What bits of your life are going okay at the moment?". Two differences here to using SFP with a fully voluntary client were that I had to share some future talk that comprised of what the professionals were looking for to be reassured about future safety and that the professionals had to have a view on what constituted progress, too.

On other occasions, when someone talks about a problem, what is wanted is more implicit. It could reasonably be assumed that we are hearing about what they *don't* want, and one response might be to ask, "What do you want to be different?" or another, "Suppose things become a bit better, what would you notice?". Using the word "first" at the end of the latter question can help in starting small. These questions can be useful – and difficult to answer. It is often helpful to make a guess about what is wanted *instead* of the problem and check this with a closed question, inviting the answer "Yes". When this comes, it can have a galvanising effect, turning a conversation around from looking back at problems towards a more hoped-for future.

I was contacted by a client in crisis, a significant part of which was not knowing if he could continue in his job, having fallen out with his boss. He had seen his work as the only positive aspect of his life, which he was now worried was going to fall apart. His stuckness continually returned him to explanations of his work problems, which I was also getting caught up in, and so I was in danger of becoming stuck, too. I then asked, "Look, do you want to give it a go still, even with what has happened? Do you want to get this sorted somehow?". After he answered, "Yes", I plugged away for the next 15 minutes with two main questions, one inviting future talk – *How would you notice on your next day at work that it is on the way to being sorted?* (with its built-in follow-up: *How else?*) – and the other, progress talk – *What do you know about yourself – and your boss – that tells you that you can get it sorted?*

Ending

Almost by definition, it is not easy to plan how to end unplanned SF conversations. You might need to return to the other aspects of your job within which you have used parts of the SF approach. If you will meet again and have invited your client to engage in progress talk, you could say that you will be interested to hear about any other progress they notice when you see them next. If future talk has been more predominant, you could ask them to notice any of those things they have spoken about happening. I wished my client with work problems well, and when I saw him next, I decided to see whether we could restart an SF conversation by checking if I might ask him about any progress he had noticed, to which he replied, "Yes".

References

de Shazer, S., Berg, I. K., Lipchik, E., Nunnally, E., Molnar, A., Gingerich, W., & Weiner-Davis, M. (1986). Brief therapy: Focused solution development. *Family Process*, *25*(2), 207–221. https://doi.org/10.1111/j.1545–5300.1986.00207.x.

Ellmann, R. (1982). *James Joyce* (2nd ed.). Oxford University Press.

Fisher, R., Ury, W., & Patton, B. (2011). *Getting to yes* (3rd ed.). Penguin Books.

Gingerich, W., de Shazer, S., & Weiner-Davis, M. (1988). Constructing change: A research view of interviewing. In E. Lipchik (ed.), *Interviewing* (pp. 21–32). Aspen.

Hopwood, L., & de Shazer, S. (2021). From here to there to who knows where: The continuing evolution of solution-focused brief therapy. *Journal of Solution Focused Practices*, *5*(1), Article 9. https://digitalscholarship.unlv.edu/cgi/viewcontent.cgi?article=1118&context=journalsfp Accessed 24 September 2024.

Isebaert, L. (2017). *Solution-focused cognitive and systemic therapy*. Routledge.

Larkin, P. (1990). For Sidney Bechet. In *Collected poems* (p. 83). Faber & Faber.

O'Hanlon, B., & Beadle, S. (1996). *A field guide to possibility land*. BT Press.

Shennan, G. (2019). *Solution focused practice: Effective communication to facilitate change* (2nd ed.). Red Globe Press.

Shennan, G., & Iveson, C. (2011). From solution to description: Practice and research in tandem. In C. Franklin, T. Trepper, W. Gingerich, & E. McCollum (eds.), *Solution-focused brief therapy: A handbook of evidence-based practice* (pp. 281–298). Oxford University Press.

Unwin, D. (2005). SFGP! Why a solution focused approach is brilliant in primary care. *Solution News*, *1*(4), 10–12.

Weakland, J., Fisch, R., Watzlawick, P., & Bodin, A. (1974). Brief therapy: Focused problem resolution. *Family Process*, *13*(2), 141–168. https://doi.org/10.1111/j.1545–5300.1974.00141.x.

Chapter 5

Solution Focused Practice in UK mental health settings – where next?

Evan George

In 1987, Chris Iveson, Harvey Ratner and I were working in a North London systemically oriented community Mental Health Service, and all of us were also teaching Systemic Psychotherapy at the Institute of Family Therapy (London) when, somewhat by chance, we came across Solution Focused Brief Therapy (SFBT) and the work of Steve de Shazer and his colleagues in Milwaukee. Reading the book (de Shazer, 1985), there was just one book at the time, and all the early papers that the Milwaukee team had published, left us intrigued and fascinated, curious and excited but also, understandably, a little sceptical. How could this approach work, an approach which seemed to challenge so many of our rooted assumptions about the practice of therapy and if it did work, how likely were the changes to be maintained? However, our excitement outweighed our doubts, and we set up a project, the Brief Therapy Project, to test the model (as it then was back in 1987) with a wide range of clients referred to a service that rather unusually worked with children and families, adolescents, adults and older people, and worked across the full range of community mental health referrals. Very soon, we saw that despite having had no training in SFBT, our attempts to practice the approach, based merely on our reading, seemed to work in the sense that a very wide range of clients were reporting change. Our excitement, interest and curiosity grew, and our scepticism began to abate – slowly.

In 1987, when we set about learning SFBT, there were no training courses in the UK. Indeed, the only course of which we were aware was a month's practicum in Milwaukee. Being unable to take up this opportunity, both for financial reasons and owing to family commitments, we considered how else we could take our 'self-training' forward; so, in 1989, we invited Steve de Shazer to come to London to present his work and to consult to our team. His visit in 1990, when he was accompanied by his partner Insoo Kim Berg, was the first of a series of regular visits which lasted until his death in 2005.

Following the success of his first visit and the interest that it elicited, we arranged a large London conference in 1992 for him to share his newest thinking and latest practice. On this occasion, he showed a teaching tape, a first session, entitled 'Coming Through the Ceiling'.[1] The client indicated that her desired outcome from her work with de Shazer was to be able to sleep, and the session

DOI: 10.4324/9781003519225-5

focused on her sleeping, with a particular interest in times when she was more able to sleep, the exceptions to the rule of the 'non-sleeping' problem (de Shazer, 1985). In passing and in a slightly embarrassed way, the client touched upon her theory about the cause of her sleeping issues, namely the presence of a neighbour living in the apartment above her who, she explained, was beaming down rays into her bedroom from a machine that he had constructed. de Shazer continued to focus on sleeping. At the end of the session, there was a degree of uproar in the room. A significant number of mental health professionals were clearly un-happy – indeed, some were outraged – that de Shazer had not focused on what they regarded as the client's clear and obvious mental health difficulties to which they attached a range of diagnostic descriptions. Their disapproval of de Shazer's choice of focus was in no way alleviated by the fact that the outcome of the piece of work was good, the client achieved the changes that she was hoping for and the changes she made were associated with further beneficial changes: a positive ripple effect. de Shazer showed some of the follow-up sessions where the changes that he claimed were clear and evident. However, the fact that de Shazer had not focused, at least directly in a way that they could understand, on what this group of sceptics regarded as the underlying problem – the client's mental health condition – was difficult for them to accept.

The puzzlement of this group of mental health professionals back in 1992 is still in evidence, albeit to a somewhat lesser extent, today. The world of mental healthcare, operating within the medical model, has in the past been significantly dominated by concepts of formulation, diagnosis and assessment. The need to fig-ure out what is 'really' going on and what is causing it to go on has tended to be viewed as the only valid foundation for treatment and as the gateway to services.

The idea that we can work successfully with clients without knowing anything about the problem which brings them to us both was, and in some contexts remains, hard to understand for many professionals working in mental health services. de Shazer's work was truly revolutionary, questioning the very bases of generally ac-cepted practice, and it is therefore perhaps not surprising that SFBT was slower to be adopted in mental health settings than the developing evidence of effectiveness might surely have warranted.

The challenges to traditional thinking that SFBT[2] presents can be encapsu-lated in terms of two requirements: two demands that the approach makes of the practitioner, namely the need to 'trust our clients' and the need to 'believe in them'. The practitioner's choosing to trust is reflected in myriad ways in every piece of work. We ask clients what their 'best hopes' from the work are (George et al., 1999), and we choose to accept their response as the starting point for our conversation rather than choosing to know better or to know differently. We choose to trust our clients to know whom to invite to the session, and we work with whomsoever they bring. We choose to trust our clients to tell us whatever we might need to know for the work to progress. We choose to trust the client's evaluation of our work together, 'useful' or 'not useful'; and if 'not useful', it is incumbent upon us to 'do something different' (de Shazer et al., 2007). We choose to trust the client's thinking about whether it would be useful for us to meet again and to trust their thinking about how long a gap between sessions would be right for them. We choose to trust clients to find their own best ways of making progress between sessions and assume that they will; thus, there is no need to 'pin the client down', no formal action planning. At most, we might wonder which of the many ideas that the client has come up with during the course of our talking they might choose to use first or whether they might find something else to take them forward in a useful way. The choice that the Solution Focused practitioner makes to trust touches upon every aspect of our work (George, 2020a). And yet this position that we choose to take seems directly at odds with that which has come to caricature team-meeting-based conversation in mental healthcare, with clients sometimes talked about as if they cannot be expected to know what a good outcome might be, and cannot be allowed to be the arbiter regarding the effectiveness of the work; cannot be trusted to mean what they say and so on. It is the worker or team's task to peer through the surface, beneath and behind the presentation: to determine, on the basis of their own expert knowledge and training, what is 'really' going on. The worker is regarded as having privileged access to reality, an access that is denied to the client. In the Solution Focused world, on the other hand, there is no 'really'; there are merely the client's words, and it is with those words that we choose to work.

If the dominance of the medical model has made 'trusting' difficult – indeed, it has framed the idea of 'trusting' as naïve, or perhaps even unprofessional – 'believing' in our clients is equally challenging for many.

In Solution Focused Practice (SFP), believing in our clients is not an option; it is not dependent on assessment; it is a position that we choose to adopt; it is a part of the discipline of the approach (George, 2020b). When we meet a client for the first time, we can have no evidence relating to their capacity to change. We know little or nothing about them, and yet we choose to believe that they have everything necessary to be successful in achieving their best hopes from the work and having made this choice, we look for the evidence that this is indeed so, listening for resources, listening for achievements, listening for exceptions and instances (Iveson et al., 2012), listening for capacity.

Since, by and large, we hear what we listen for, what we subsequently hear 'back-fills' with evidence of our chosen assumption about the client. However, this position of believing extends further. The Solution Focused practitioner chooses to believe that every client is motivated by something and that it is our job to discover what that 'something' is. Further, we choose to believe that when the client says that they want to change, they indeed mean it (Ratner et al., 2012).

Insoo Kim Berg describes this position as follows:

It is assumed that the client is competent to know what is good for her and her family. It is further assumed that the client has the ability to solve problems and has solved problems in the past.

(Berg, 1994, p. 61)

Since every client is assumed to be giving their best to collaborate with the change process, whatever form their best might take, there is no place within the model for the concept of client-based resistance (de Shazer, 1984). Letting go of this concept, which underpins so much traditional thinking in mental health services, is difficult, demanding and disorienting. It might, therefore, be argued that rather than being surprised that the approach has not been more widely adopted, given the extent to which Solution Focused Practice diverges from traditional mental health practice, perhaps we should be more surprised that the approach has been adopted as much as it has. If this is the case, how should we explain this significant adoption of the approach substantially against the odds?

Perhaps we should start by acknowledging that the context for 'therapeutic interventions' has changed considerably since the 1980s. There is a much broader acceptance of the utility of brief interventions and of interventions that are not 'insight-oriented'. Indeed, in many settings, single-session consultations or 'one-at-a-time' work is the offering of choice. In addition, the increasing interest in neuroscience and in particular in the concept of neuroplasticity, as well as a growing focus on resilience and survival, have together supported the emergence of a more hopeful outlook, challenging the limiting impact of such ideas as 'damage' and inviting us to think instead about recovery and adaptation. Further, the emergence of SFBT has coincided with a period of increased scepticism regarding Grand Theories generally and of a rather belated challenge to the manner in which the experiences, life preferences, beliefs and values of minority groups generally have been obscured and subsequently ignored within so many approaches to therapy. It is within this context that Solution Focused Practice, which treats each session as if it could be the last and assumes that each session should aspire to be useful, which typically offers open-ended interventions but averages three to five sessions, which centres on the client, their best hopes (rather than our diagnosis) and their best way of making progress (rather than our solutions), can and should be able to thrive.

Just as the macro context within which Solution Focused practitioners find themselves working has changed over the past 40 years, so, too, has the micro. Demand has increased, and waiting lists have lengthened, whether in Adult or Child and Adolescent services; an increase fuelled, at least in part, by the Covid-19 pandemic, which has also driven the necessity to find new and innovative ways of delivering for services users.

We now see Solution Focused Practice being successfully delivered face-to-face, of course, but also on the phone, online, by text, in chatrooms and even by email. This flexibility of delivery is matched by the range of 'homes for conversation' that practitioners have found to be amenable to the approach: formal appointments through to in-passing corridor interactions; out-patient work and in-patient work; review meetings, group-work and couple-work; mentoring, supervision, consultation and conflict resolution; team coaching and organisational interventions. In all of these 'settings', SFP has been put to work and has proved its worth. Yet, the approach's flexibility extends further: the Solution Focused approach can justifiably be used with any referral no matter what the 'problem' might be. This obviates the necessity for a 'therapeutic' assessment at the beginning of an intervention. The Solution Focused worker can just get on with it, whatever the presentation, and expects to make a difference from the first meeting onwards. Once the worker has decided that a change-oriented intervention is 'viable', that immediate attention to the client's safety is not required (although, as Michele Orr argues in this book, at that time, too), then the approach can be used, and since the intervention is likely to be relatively short, more clients can be seen.

Of course, in a context of risk, our role and responsibility might legitimate us, indeed might require us, to pursue a focus that is not derived solely from the client's 'best hopes' but also from our concerns about the client's welfare. However, even here, the conversation will be transformed by our appreciative, 'trusting' and 'believing' stance. This stance might lead us, for example, to enquire about occasions in the past when the client has come through crises well and safely and invite us to be interested in how they have done that, what has worked for them and of all the things that have worked what is most likely to be useful to them in this situation. We might ask the client to think about the qualities and capacities that they have drawn on to help them to keep going in the past when life was difficult and invite them to be curious about what difference it might make if they were drawing on those self-same capacities now. We might ask about who, of all the significant persons in their life, past or present, would be most confident that they can get through this crisis and what this person, or those people, know about the client that gives them confidence. We might be curious about who is most concerned about them at present and what the smallest changes would be that that person would need to see for them to be convinced that the client can keep themselves safe. And even if there are issues that the worker is obliged to address (as part of any statutory responsibilities), we can be open about this, 'I am going to have to talk with you about X even though I know that you would prefer not to, and while I am talking with you about X what could you get out of this conversation that might make it useful to you – even a little bit?'. This 'twin-tracking' (Ratner et al., 2012) has the advantage of openness and transparency whilst also acknowledging that the client may have their own legitimate 'best hopes' for the conversation. Addressing both 'agendas' in a meeting is likely to be more engaging for the client than merely pursuing the professional agenda. However, it is important to add that whilst the Solution Focused practitioner's stance is one of appreciation and trust, our trust is not blind when it comes to risk assessments. If we ask the client what it is that gives them so much confidence that they can keep themselves safe, whilst, of course, we will be interested in the answer, in relation to safety, we must be convinced: there will have to be evidence. In relation to safety, we cannot 'delegate' our decision to the client entirely, however much we respect their view and believe in their capacity to change.

The increased interest in Solution Focused Practice within UK mental health-care may also have been supported by a further characteristic of the approach which might be described as its impact on client and worker alike. The impact on the client is striking. When observing sessions, it is not unusual to notice changes in body posture and eye contact and to hear changes in voice tone, all of which might reasonably be considered the external manifestations of clients feeling better about themselves. Engaging in Solution Focused conversations appears to increase a sense of hopefulness, possibility and optimism. It also appears to be associated with an increased sense of self-efficacy and agency, with clients typically owning the changes made – 'I did it!'. Since each session appears to impact positively on the client, building their sense of self-worth, Solution Focused interventions are 'non-disruptive' (George, 2023) in client's lives and clients, therefore, are not required to be in a good-enough place prior to starting work. This effect was more than clear at the end of a first family meeting[3] when the father in the family, as he was standing up to leave, punched the air twice and exclaimed, 'We can do it, we can do it!'. Interestingly, the family cancelled the next session, stating that they now knew that they could move forward positively without further meetings.

This impact on the client is mirrored by the impact on the worker. Workers in public health services in the UK, certainly since the time of the pandemic, have described themselves as feeling overworked, tired, under-appreciated and under-supported. However, practitioners who adopt the Solution Focused approach not unusually comment on the work feeling lighter, less burdensome, more enjoyable and more rewarding. Just as clients typically appreciate noticing changes relatively quickly, so too do workers. And as Medina and Beyebach (2014) have convincingly argued – and as will Aine Garvey later in this book – Solution Focused Practice seems to protect workers against burnout. This way of working seems to be as good for the worker as it is for the client. Sessions are fun, and there is often a great deal of smiling, indeed, of laughing, even when the client has attended to address tough and painful issues. It may be that the influence of the unhelpful aphorism 'no pain, no gain', which has cast such a deep shadow over the practice of therapy, is at last being challenged. Therapeutic pain is the therapist's choice, not a necessity or an inevitability (George, 2023).

Despite the extent to which Solution Focused Practice might not always be a comfortable fit with those mental health practices still organised by the medical model, the changing context – the increase in demand following Covid, the flexibility of the approach and the positive impact that this way of working has both on client and worker – all go some way towards explaining its adoption.

As we look to the future, there are a number of additional changes in the culture of mental healthcare delivery, some of which are already happening of course, that could be seen as the required context for Solution Focus to take a more central position in everyday mental health practice and which in turn would be amplified by the increasing adoption of the model:

1   It is likely that we will be seeing an increasing 'relativisation' regarding the concept of 'diagnosis'. Diagnosis would come to be viewed as merely a construct, one way of thinking about people, which can be useful in some contexts but is not 'true'; merely an attempt to categorise certain patterns of behaviour and to describe them. As diagnosis becomes appreciated as just one way of organising our interventions, we would be more focused on the questions 'What does the

client want?' and 'How will the client know that our work has been useful?'. The client's voice and the client's preference will be more central in our work.

2   We are likely also to see greater professional humility. As Berg and Szabo write, 'There is no real understanding of what others really want to tell us. There are only more useful misunderstandings and less useful misunderstandings' (2005, p. 127). And in the words of Eve Lipchik, we will recognise that 'You cannot change clients they can only change themselves' (2002, p. 17). All we can do is create the context within which that change happens.

3   We will be letting go of our certainty, moving to a position of conscious and determined 'not-knowing' as Anderson and Goolishian at the Galveston Institute (Anderson & Goolishian, 1992) advocate, adopting instead of 'knowing' a position of inquiry, asking questions which allow the client to chart their own path forward. 'Asking' will take the place of telling, which is of particular importance when we are encountering people from minoritised groups and where anti-oppressive ways of working are of particular importance.

4   The growth of Solution Focused Practice will fit with a changed way of thinking about clients: a choice to focus on clients' strengths and skills, unique talents and resources, rather than their deficits and limitations.

5   The wider adoption of Solution Focused Practice will be associated with all of us learning to talk differently about our clients – even behind their backs – perhaps choosing to mirror the BRIEF team's commitment only ever to talk about clients as if they can hear every word that we say. The way that we talk about clients impacts on the way that we think about clients, and the way that we think about clients impacts on the way that we interact with them.

6   And finally, the mental health field will be moving away from ideas of treatment and management to ideas of service. We will be focused on serving our clients, who are, after all, the most important people in our professional lives.

Notes

1   Coming through the Ceiling is a reconstruction of a recorded two-session therapy using an actor as the client with Steve de Shazer as himself, the therapist.

2   When referring to the model that de Shazer and team developed, I refer to it as Solution Focused Brief Therapy (SFBT). When referring to the way that the approach is being utilised across a wide range of settings in the UK, many of which are not primarily therapeutic, I refer to Solution Focused Practice (SFP).

3   This was a therapy with a reconstituted family who brought four children to the session. The therapist was Evan George.

References

Anderson, H., & Goolishian, H. (1992). The client is the expert: A not-knowing approach to therapy. In S. McNamee, & K. J. Gergen (eds.), *Therapy as social construction* (pp. 25–39). Sage Publications, Inc.

Berg, I. K. (1994). *Family based services: A solution-focused approach*. Norton.

Berg, I. K., & Szabo, P. (2005). *Brief coaching for lasting solutions*. Norton.

de Shazer, S. (1984). The death of resistance. *Family Process, 23*, 11–21, The death of Resistance 1984 (solutions-centre.org).

de Shazer, S. (1985). *Keys to solution in brief therapy*. Norton.

de Shazer, S., Dolan, Y., Korman, H., Trepper, T., MacCollum, E., & Berg, I. K. (2007). *More than Miracles: The state of the art of solution focused therapy*. Haworth.

George, E. (2020a). *Trust*. www.brief.org.uk/blog/trust.html.

George, E. (2020b). *Trusting or believing or trusting and believing*. www.brief.org.uk/blog/trusting-or-believing-or-trusting-and-believing.html.

George, E. (2023). *Therapeutic distress is optional – not necessary or inevitable*. www.brief.org.uk/blog/therapeutic-distress-is-optional-not-necessary-or-inevitable.html.

George, E., Iveson, C., and Ratner, H. (1990). *Problem to solution: Brief therapy with individuals and families* (Revised & expanded ed. 1999). BT Press.

Iveson, C., George, E., & Ratner, H. (2012). *Brief coaching: A solution focused approach*. Routledge.

Lipchik, E. (2002). *Beyond technique in solution-focused therapy*. Guildford.

Medina, A., & Beyebach, M. (2014). The impact of solution-focused training on professionals' beliefs, practices and burnout of child protection workers in Tenerife Island. *Child Care in Practice, 20*(1), 7–36. https://doi.org/10.1080/13575279.2013.847058.

Ratner, H., George, E., & Iveson, C. (2012). *Solution focused brief therapy: 100 Key ideas and techniques*. Routledge.

Chapter 6

'This magical lightbulb went off in my head' – How training NHS staff in Solution Focused Practice can change the experience of people presenting in mental health crisis

Rose McCabe, Aamena Akubat, Alexandra E. Bakou and Maria Long

In this chapter, we will describe experiences of delivering a brief Solution Focused intervention to young people and adults following a presentation to the Emergency Department (ED)[1] with self-harm and/or suicidality. We describe experiences from two research trials underway in the UK. The ASSURED study is recruiting 620 adults across several hospitals in London, Devon and the Midlands (Improving outcomes in clients who self-harm – Adapting and evaluating a brief psychological intervention in Emergency Departments: https://assuredstudy.co.uk). The SASH study is recruiting 144 young people aged 12–18 (Supporting Adolescents with Self-Harm: https://sashstudy.co.uk). Both studies are randomised controlled trials comparing therapeutic assessment, enhanced safety planning and Solution Focused sessions with usual care.

We will discuss how the SFP intervention differs from usual care, who is delivering the sessions and ongoing supervision; present three case studies involving clients from minoritised/marginalised groups; show how Solution Focused questions uncover new information about resources and capabilities; and present feedback from mental health practitioners newly trained in Solution Focused Practice (SFP), along with young people and adults on their experience of Solution Focused sessions.

Why have we chosen this approach?

As has been explained in previous chapters, Solution Focused Brief Therapy (SFBT) is a strengths-based approach focusing on the client's best hopes for the future. Many clients who present in crisis with self-harm and/or suicidal thoughts find it difficult to imagine a better and brighter future. Consistent with Adam S. Froerer's views earlier in the book, most other talking therapies offered in the NHS, such as Trauma-Informed Therapy or Cognitive/Dialectical Behavioural Therapy

DOI: 10.4324/9781003519225-6

usually focus on past experiences, problems and difficulties. In contrast, SFBT supports the client in recognising their best hopes and highlights what is already working, along with the person's strengths and resources. It has the potential to instil hope in patients who present with suicidal thoughts (Henden, 2017). In a comprehensive review, Jerome et al. (2023) have synthesised how Solution Focused (SF) approaches have been conceptualised and understood within the adult mental health literature. Here, we talk about Solution Focused Practice because it describes how the practitioners in both studies are working: they are often not therapists per se, and they are working in teams where SF approaches are not routinely implemented.

How are the ASSURED/SASH interventions different from usual care?

There are around 220,000 contacts for self-harm in EDs in England annually (Cooper et al., 2015). A psychosocial assessment in the ED aims to assess the patients' risk, needs for care and a management plan. While people who self-harm often require further support, several barriers delay access to appropriate services: lack of service availability (McCarthy et al., 2024), long waiting lists, high thresholds for entry to specialist mental health services and services not accepting clients as they are deemed too high risk (Quinlivan et al., 2023).

ASSURED and SASH offer rapid follow-up support within around two weeks of attending the ED. Four sessions are offered to adults (with an optional bank session) and up to eight sessions for young people and carers. Usually, when a young person is in crisis, parents/carers are also going through a difficult time. The first session following ED attendance involves a therapeutic assessment and enhanced safety planning. The subsequent sessions are Solution Focused sessions. Sessions are offered either face-to-face (with some crisis Child and Adolescent Mental Health Services (CAMHS) requiring this) or by video call or phone call.

While our studies suggest a timeline for sessions, with increasing intervals between sessions, these can be flexibly arranged with the person. In ASSURED, four sessions are offered: at around Week 1, Week 2, Week 4 and Week 8, with an optional bank session over a nine-month period. In SASH, up to six sessions are offered: at Week 1, Week 2, Week 4 and Week 8, with two optional sessions over the subsequent three months. Two additional optional sessions are offered to parents or carers. These are face-to-face or remote sessions, depending on preference/the requirements of the service. There is flexibility, with a recent session delivered on a ward after a young person was hospitalised due to self-harm. There are opportunities to rearrange following session non-attendance, which has supported engagement and more positive experiences of support. Flexibility in arranging the sessions to meet the person/ young person/family where they are and around other commitments has been important for fostering rapport and maintaining engagement. Also, allowing for some non-attendance at sessions and not "discharging" people has been very important, as people may still be in crisis and find it difficult to attend sessions as planned.

Practitioners delivering the intervention and supervision

Staffing and staff mix varies across our study sites. Hence, we have trained a range of practitioners with different professional backgrounds and levels of experience. We have trained around 130 mental health practitioners working in Psychiatric Liaison teams in EDs and Crisis CAMHS teams (NHS roles at Band 6 or 7) along with assistant psychologists (Band 5), support workers, family therapists, associate clinical psychologists and doctors doing postgraduate training in psychiatry. Training is for two days, with access to online videos, a manual and suggested scripts.

For most practitioners, SFP is a major paradigm shift from their usual way of working. As a result, supervision has been particularly important for our aspiration to provide as pure a version of Solution Focused Practice as possible and to ensure the wellbeing of practitioners working in a new way with people presenting with self-harm and suicidality. Practitioners are encouraged to attend weekly group supervision, which has been particularly important early on when practitioners are trying out SFP for the first time. Supervision involves discussion of cases, noticing what has gone well and collaborative problem-solving when attempting to work in a Solution Focused way within the NHS context (e.g., especially around risk management) and reviewing session transcripts/videos where available. In their usual practice, practitioners working in EDs and Crisis CAMHS teams have been more likely to have monthly supervision due to the busyness of these environments.

Case studies

The following three case studies involve people who either reported discrimination or are more likely to have experienced discrimination associated with various protected characteristics, including their ethnic identity, sexual identity, neurodiversity and residence status in the UK. Their identities have been anonymised.

Naomi (they/them)

Naomi is a 45-year-old White Irish person who identifies as gender neutral and who presented to the ED following long-term attempts to access gender reassignment surgery from their GP. Their GP informed them that they would need to undergo therapy prior to being offered breast removal surgery. Naomi had undergone several therapies offered by the NHS and found none to be beneficial. They expressed feeling "extremely uncomfortable within [their] own skin" and couldn't imagine continuing to live without undergoing surgery to remove their breasts. This continued to increase their suicidal thoughts as Naomi reported "constant discrimination" and "receiving conditional care" after feeling deceived by their GP. Upon joining the research study, they expressed this being their "last hope" before taking active measures to end their life. Naomi engaged in Solution Focused conversations and was able to explore their best hopes of living with or without gender reassignment surgery. Through asking the miracle question: visualising living with or without surgery as well as the difference this would make in their life, Naomi moved from describing panic attacks and nightmares, which they felt would only end after surgery, to small signs of progress. These included not being stressed, having a routine and spending more time outside of their home. Naomi described what they would want to feel instead of panic/nightmares about their future: contentment in their day, a day that was in their control.

Naomi discussed difficult past experiences with professionals that had deeply impacted their trust. In previous therapeutic/clinical relationships, they encountered inconsistencies, unfulfilled promises and a lack of empathy, which led them to feel vulnerable and betrayed. Naomi often approached each session with caution, hesitant to open up fully due to fear of being let down or misunderstood. The first session took place over the phone. The second session was held online and the third session was in person, which had the greatest impact. The practitioner reflected:

> They were able to see myself in a physical form as the clinical practitioner sitting before them and displaying an eagerness to support them through this difficult time . . . barriers were gradually broken down and Naomi ended the sessions feeling hopeful of a positive future.

Stephen

Stephen is a 26-year-old male from Albania. He fled his country following altercations with a local gang and fear of harm to his life. Stephen sought asylum in the UK due to the threats to his life. The court hearings and asylum process increased his anxieties and low mood. He had minimal support within the UK, as his friends and family remained in Albania. However, he developed a good relationship with his flatmate. Stephen presented to the ED after an overdose due to fear of being returned to Albania. In his Solution Focused sessions, asking the miracle question allowed him to explore what difference asylum might make to him. Although the verdict was completely out of the control of the client and practitioner, both explored how Stephen would be able to continue to maintain hope through this difficult time. Unfortunately, his asylum application was rejected.

Despite this, Stephen surprised himself. He directed his energy into the gym to gain physical and mental benefit instead of becoming self-destructive, as he had expected. Stephen acknowledged that although he had no control over his immigration status, he had control of his emotions and responses and, therefore, was able to maintain composure and practice his coping mechanisms. This, in turn, led Stephen to end the Solution Focused intervention "being positive" and "seeking joy in living life for what it is", which was a huge contrast with the first session soon after attending the ED. What follows is a brief excerpt from the session with Stephen just after his asylum application had been rejected. Questions are asked (emboldened in the text, with added commentary) which support the client to focus on how he has responded well to bad news and who has noticed:

Practitioner: So considering the outcome you received from the court . . . **Did you surprise yourself in the way you responded?** *[Rather than focusing on the bad news and how difficult this was, this question focuses on how the client responded in a positive way and encourages elaboration of his coping]*

Stephen: Yeah, really, because to be honest, I was very, very . . . I didn't expect this response, to be honest. I was hoping for something better.

Practitioner: Yeah.

Stephen: I wasn't expecting this, but, yeah, it's gone good, you know?

Practitioner: Yes?

Stephen: Because I have controlled myself.

Some lines of the transcript are omitted here.

Practitioner: Yeah. **So you were surprised and pleased about how you actually were able to control yourself?** *[This "so" prefaced formulation encourages elaboration on how the client managed to control himself]*

Stephen: Yeah.

Practitioner: Good, good. Really good. Well done. Um, okay . . . **So you said, like, the things that have been working for you are going for walks. Have you been doing anything else to keep yourself feeling better?** *[Here, the practitioner refers to what's working for the client. They add a closed question. This is actually a no-inviting question through the use of the word anything. It could have been more open, e.g., What else have you been doing to keep yourself feeling better?]*

Stephen: On a couple of days, not much, really. Not much . . . but trying to.

Practitioner: Have you still been talking to your friends and family?

Stephen: Yes.

Practitioner: Okay. Okay. **And has anything happened recently to give you hope that things could be the way you'd like them to be?** *[As with the previous, this is a closed, no-inviting question. It could have been more open, e.g., What else has happened that gives you hope that things can get better?]*

Stephen: No, not really.

Practitioner: What about the fact that you've got the option to appeal the case?

Stephen: Yeah, that's the only thing. That's the only hope, like, I'm having for the moment.

Practitioner: Okay. **And then, so who do you think has noticed these changes in you? In the fact that you were able to control yourself; in the fact that you were still talking to your friends and family, which you might otherwise not have; the fact that you're**

	still going for walks; the fact that you're cooking; the fact that you're coming to these sessions. **Who do you think has noticed?** *[This question draws attention to the positive strategies the client has been using and invites an "other person perspective", which is a key technique of SFP]*
Stephen:	The friend I live with.
Practitioner:	Okay. **And how do you think he might have noticed?** *[This question asks the client to describe what the client's friend has noticed to highlight the client's actions]*
Stephen:	Because he knows me before I try to suicide myself, and he knows all my problems. That's why, you know, he keeps saying, "You need to be strong. You need to do this".
Practitioner:	Yeah. **And do you think he's pleased by . . .** *[This carries the assumption and draws attention to the client's friend being pleased by his way of coping with his challenging situation]*
Stephen:	Yeah.
Practitioner:	Yeah. **And how do you know that he has noticed?** *[This interactional question seeks to unpack what the client's friend has noticed and highlight any small actions that might show coping]*
Stephen:	I know because he has been telling me.
Practitioner:	He's been telling you.
Stephen:	Yeah. He tells me. He tells me, like, "You're doing good; you're doing this!", you know?
Practitioner:	You are doing good. Okay. **And what difference do you feel that makes to you?** *[This draws attention to the client's desired outcome]*
Stephen:	It makes for me a big difference because it's like, I'm doing something good for myself, you know? I'm doing the right thing.
Practitioner:	Yeah, absolutely. Okay. **And how do you think you are able to continue these changes?** *[This strategy question explores and assumes that the client will be able to continue with the changes he has made]*
Stephen:	I just feel like I don't want to give up, you know?
Practitioner:	Yeah.
Stephen:	I'm keeping hope, like. Yeah, kept hope, 'til I have a chance, you know?

At the beginning of the sessions, Stephen was in crisis, having made a serious attempt on his life. Stephen recently moved to the UK, and while he was trying to settle in, he'd been struggling with overwhelming feelings, including thoughts of suicide. Adjusting to a new environment had brought challenges and emotions that were difficult for him to manage alone. He came to all sessions and used the bank session, as he felt that the therapy could help him understand these feelings and develop strategies to cope. Between and during sessions, he identified further signs of coping and progress.

Ariel

Ariel is a 30-year-old Black British female of Caribbean descent. She has a learning disability and is determined that this will not hold her back in how she experiences the world and opportunities. Ariel described feeling "up and down" and "having periods of hypermania" and intervals of "depression", but also "feeling confident, sociable, driven and having a positive outlook on life".

Ariel describes a loving support network, particularly her mother, grandmother and a best friend, who resides overseas. Although Ariel describes these relationships as nurturing, she expresses "feeling criticised", and her loved ones believing that she "constantly be seeking attention". In her workplace, Ariel has had numerous difficulties with her manager's lack of understanding about her learning disability and expects her "disability to be sorted and cured by October through therapy". Ariel has found the lack of empathy from her place of work and home environment difficult to manage, leading to a suicide attempt.

Ariel has outlined her best hopes as: managing emotions better, increasing self-esteem and talking about challenging situations. Ariel has reflected on occasions in which she felt she was being hard on herself. During the Solution Focused sessions, Ariel has decided she would be: "putting myself first and making myself happy, feel more confident in myself, trusting myself to do great things!".

Ariel attended all four of the sessions offered to her. She had previously undergone other therapies in the NHS and privately. She mentioned "always finding [therapy] helpful" and dived deep into SF sessions with the intention to benefit as far as possible. Ariel requested longer intervals between sessions to extend the time being supported. Her sessions were spread over 16 weeks as opposed to 12 weeks. Ariel went on her first solo trip whilst participating in the intervention; she was able to utilise the session prior to her departure to discuss her best hopes for her travels and what she hoped to achieve throughout the journey. On her return, a further session was able to review what had gone well.

Practitioners' and clients' perspectives; changes in ways of working and wellbeing

Using SFP has been reported to be a different experience by practitioners whose usual focus is risk management and case management. Medina and Beyebach (2014) found that social workers who were trained in SFP – and particularly those who changed their practice in the direction of becoming more collaborative – were less likely to suffer from burnout. We will be exploring this systematically in our studies.

Before being trained in SFP, practitioners were mostly not aware of the model. After training, while many described being very positive about the opportunity and the potential of SFP to improve outcomes, they also had reservations:

> At first, I wasn't sure about it . . . just compared to what I'm usually doing, which is very problem-focused . . . and the population are quite traumatised . . . I had

reservations that it would be invalidating by not focusing on the negative . . . and whether the young person would be OK with just focusing on where they want to be . . . but then I think over time with this young person it's worked very well . . . between the first and second session I was surprised by the shift that had occurred.

Practitioners have described noticing how SFP creates a shift in the conversation from the past to the future whilst continuing to validate past experiences. This is different to other therapies currently available in the NHS and empowers clients to leave the intervention hopeful for their future.

Clients describe coming up with the answers themselves because of the questions asked, along with recognising they are strong and have control over how they view situations:

And then it was like this magical light bulb went off in my head . . . I can see what I've done. I can see what I've accomplished. I can see what I've achieved. I can see how I feel differently now. And it's not just because I was given a straight-up answer, because I was made to find the answer within myself because of the questions . . . . Because the answer is always within ourselves . . . . So, having that type of person available to you . . . that was a big help and that shifted everything.
I am really strong, I have the ability to open up and things can change for me.
. . . and being able to have some sense of control of the way I view a particular situation [is really important for me].

A young person working with us on SASH said:

I was so happy that the intervention is being rolled out and is now making a tangible difference to young people in crisis . . . . If the intervention was around when I was in crisis, I know I would have felt so supported by it . . . . [It] truly will make such a big impact.

Practitioners have described Solution Focused sessions with young people as being more playful and less onerous than comparable sessions of CBT, where homework is expected and might be difficult to negotiate around school commitments. Practitioners found identifying points of connection between young people and their parents' best hopes for their child can provide a basis for improvement in relationships which are often strained. Given that relationship problems between family members are among the most commonly reported problems in adolescents who self-harm (Hawton et al., 2012), this may contribute to a reduction in the risk of repeated self-harm.

Does Solution Focused Practice support anti-discrimination?

Many of the people presenting with self-harm in these studies also have a diagnosis of borderline personality disorder or complex emotional needs. They often have poor experiences of care and face stigma from practitioners as they can frequently present to the ED in crisis. Many fall between the gaps in services. Hence, they do not receive sufficient support in the community, leading to cyclical crisis presentations. Staff find this challenging, and these clients are often referred to as "manipulative" and "attention seeking", with practitioners feeling powerless to help them (O'Keeffe et al., 2021). Unfortunately, in the ED, people presenting with self-harm often report negative experiences and their distress is not taken seriously or is implicitly undermined or challenged. These responses from practitioners can be used to justify decisions not to provide further support or referrals to specialist services (Bergen et al., 2023).

In SFP, there is no role for diagnosis, which removes labels and assumptions about clients. This is of interest to many in mental health services who are of the view that diagnosis should not play such a significant role (e.g., Kendell & Jablensky, 2003). This holds for many labels, which bring with them assumptions about competence and resources, including ethnic and cultural identity, gender and sexual identity, as well as people dependent on substances and homeless people. As the practitioner's stance is one of belief in clients, it is a fundamentally hopeful way of working. Solution Focused questions come from a place of "not knowing", which is very different to a psychiatric focus on assessment, diagnosis and formulation of the problem. Practitioners stay very close to the client's own words and echo these in subsequent questions. This helps people feel listened to, taken seriously and believed. The focus on the client as the expert on their own life is very different to many mental health interactions where professional expertise is given prominence. Together, these principles offer a very different kind of experience for clients.

Helping newly trained SF practitioners to embed the approach

As with any new way of working, helping newly trained SF practitioners to embed the approach into their work and the work of their team requires support. Here are some of the things we have found might be helpful to others:

- A senior team leader (manager or consultant psychiatrist) who is supportive and sees the value of SFP is particularly helpful and means junior colleagues are less fearful of trying out a very different approach
- A regular supervision space so people can bring cases and discuss challenges (e.g., how to support people who are on waiting lists or navigating referrals in the mental health system) has been key
- Top-up training that can be arranged flexibly around each individual's availability
- A smartphone group where people can ask questions, share successes and also see if someone is around for a call if they would like advice or to debrief
- Having a buddy and strong peer support so people feel comfortable to practice skills or try out a role play prior to a potentially tricky session

- Attempting to align SFP with existing frameworks and procedures within the organisation, e.g., psychosocial assessments or risk assessment protocols
- Celebrating successes when using SFP by sharing feedback from clients/families through team meetings/forums, newsletters or online chats/smartphone groups
- Easy access to resources such as manuals, scripts, articles and websites that practitioners can refer to when they need support or inspiration
- Seeking and receiving feedback on SFP in the context in which people are working, allowing for continuous improvement and adaptation
- Involving clients in the process by encouraging them to share their feedback on the model, reinforcing the collaborative nature of the approach
- Encouraging practitioners to reflect on their experiences of SF methods through journaling or group discussions, helping to consolidate their learning.

Conclusion

Offering Solution Focused sessions to young people and adults following ED attendance for self-harm and/or suicidality is eminently feasible (as Michele Orr will also write about later in this book). This is a significant shift from the usual offer in the NHS and we will be exploring wider implementation and scaling up of this way of working in crisis care. Whilst we will test whether it is cost-effective in due course (and assess a range of outcomes), practitioners report that they enjoy using this approach and many clients report benefits from being supported in this way.

Note

1 Emergency Departments (EDs) are hospital departments which provide 24/7 care for serious injuries and life-threatening emergencies. Crisis and liaison mental health services work in the ED to support the mental health needs of people who present in crisis after any physical health needs are addressed.

References

Bergen, C., Bortolotti, L., Temple, R. K., Fadashe, C., Lee, C., Lim, M., & McCabe, R. (2023). Implying implausibility and undermining versus accepting peoples' experiences of suicidal ideation and self-harm in Emergency Department psychosocial assessments. *Frontiers in Psychiatry, 14*. https://doi.org/10.3389/fpsyt.2023.1197512.

Cooper, J., Steeg, S., Gunnell, D., Webb, R., Hawton, K., Bennewith, O., House, A., & Kapur, N. (2015). Variations in the hospital management of self-harm and patient outcome: A multi-site observational study in England. *Journal of Affective Disorders, 174*, 101–105. https://doi.org/10.1016/j.jad.2014.11.037.

Hawton, K., Bergen, H., Waters, K. Ness, J., Cooper., J., Steeg, S., Kapur, N. (2012). Epidemiology and nature of self-harm in children and adolescents: Findings from the multicentre study of self-harm in England. *European Child & Adolescent Psychiatry, 21*, 369–377. https://doi.org/10.1007/s00787-012-0269-6.

Henden, J. (2017). *Preventing suicide: The solution focused approach*. John Wiley & Sons.

Jerome, L., McNamee, P., Abdel-Halim, N., Elliot, K., & Woods, J. (2023). Solution-focused approaches in adult mental health research: A conceptual literature review and narrative synthesis. *Frontiers in Psychiatry, 14*. https://doi.org/10.3389/fpsyt.2023.1068006.

Kendell, R., & Jablensky, A. (2003). Distinguishing between the validity and utility of psychiatric diagnoses. *American Journal of Psychiatry, 160*(1), 4–12. https://doi.org/10.1176/appi.ajp.160.1.4.

McCarthy, M., McIntyre, J., Nathan, R., Ashworth, E., & Saini, P. (2024). Staff perspectives of emergency department pathways for people attending in suicidal crisis: A qualitative study. *Journal of Psychiatric and Mental Health Nursing, 31*(3), 313–324. https://doi.org/10.1111/jpm.12991.

Medina, A., & Beyebach, M. (2014). The impact of solution-focused Training on professionals' beliefs, practices and burnout of child protection workers in Tenerife Island. *Child Care in Practice, 20*(1), 7–36. https://doi.org/10.1080/13575279.2013.847058.

O'Keeffe, S., Suzuki, M., Ryan, M., Hunter, J., & McCabe, R. (2021). Experiences of care for self-harm in the emergency department: Comparison of the perspectives of patients, carers and practitioners. *BJPsych Open, 7*(5), e175. https://doi.org/10.1192/bjo.2021.1006.

Quinlivan, L., Gorman, L., Marks, S., Monaghan, E., Asmal, S., Webb, R. T., & Kapur, N. (2023). Liaison psychiatry practitioners' views on accessing aftercare and psychological therapies for patients who present to hospital following self-harm: Multi-site interview study. *BJPsych Open, 9*(2), e34. https://doi.org/10.1192/bjo.2023.2.

Chapter 7

Service users are doing it for themselves

Rayya Ghul and Mark Kilbey

Take Off is a mental health charity which is 100% led by service users in Kent, England.[1] It works to improve physical and mental wellbeing through providing peer-supported services, mainly in the form of groups which are either 'talking' or 'doing' based. All the services are designed, developed and delivered by service users on the simple principle of coming up with an idea, finding others who are willing and interested, trialling it and then testing it. This means the types of groups reflect the local service users' interests and ambitions rather than what others might decide are 'good for them'.

There is growing recognition and development of peer support systems for mental health across the spectrum of psychiatric and social services internationally (Shalaby & Agyapong, 2020). This has been developing slowly as stigma and negative perceptions of people with psychiatric diagnoses are longstanding and deeply held, even by mental health professionals. People with mental health problems continue to be the least likely social group to find work, be in a steady, long-term relationship, live in decent housing and be socially included despite increasing efforts to reduce stigma and promote mental health and wellbeing.

People with psychiatric diagnoses can be infantilised or over-protected by well-meaning professionals who see them as being vulnerable and requiring increased care and guidance. While some of this may be relevant when people are experiencing an acute mental health crisis, it can be detrimental to the recovery and dignity of the person when it becomes a more global perception. Peer support in mental health is almost always organised by or with mental health professionals, and the peer support workers tend to be recruited, trained and supervised by professionals within statutory Health and/or Social Care services.

In contrast, Take Off grew out of a local mental health service users' forum which provided input into the commissioning and provision of mental health services in Kent, and has been 100% service user-led from the outset and remains so. Rayya became a 'friend' of Take Off during its transition to offering peer support. Working at that time as a lecturer in Occupational Therapy at a local university, she was able to help Take Off access funding and training for service user organisations and acted as an educational consultant for the design of their peer support training. Rayya suggested that Take Off train their peers in 'Solution Focused Conversation'

DOI: 10.4324/9781003519225-7

(Solution Focused Practice skills used in the context of a mutually supportive conversation) to avoid the natural tendency to focus on problems when peers emulated the way that professionals spoke to them.

The training involved a short introduction followed by practice using a 'cheat sheet' of common Solution Focused questions:

What are you already doing?

- Are there any parts of your life where you are doing or did some of the things you want in the future?
- What parts of your life right now do you enjoy and want to continue or want to build on?
- Is there anything you used to do which you'd like to take up again?

What do you want to do?

- Suppose you could be doing anything you wanted in your life – what would that be?
  - What difference would that make?
  - Can you describe your ideal day?
  - What would you be doing?
  - Where would you be doing it?
  - Who would be around you and what would they be doing?

Turning negatives into positives

- *It's easy to complain and to talk about what we don't want.*
- *To turn this quickly into a Solution Focused conversation just ask:*
- What do you want to be doing **instead**?

Finding strengths and resources

- What are you good at? How do you do that?
- List 10 qualities or talents you possess that have helped you make positive change in your life, however small.
- Who supports you? What supports you?

Figure 7.1 The cheat sheet.

Readers may note that rather than beginning with a future-focused question, this more conversational use of SFP starts with exceptions. People in crisis are more likely to be able to identify something tangible they've been doing rather than the harder cognitive task of visualising the future. Unencumbered by professional training, which is almost always problem-focused, the peer support workers picked up the approach very quickly and some even said, 'Why don't doctors and nurses ask us these questions?'. Most notable in the way peers used the questions was how genuinely they responded to the tiniest sign of something positive when they asked people what they were actually doing. They found it easy and natural to praise 'just getting to the group', 'getting dressed' or 'chatting with someone'. Peers also particularly liked the power of asking 'instead' questions and were able to turn negatives around with ease as a natural part of the conversation.

Solution Focused techniques resonated with Mark, who had worked previously as a service user expert for mental health professionals. He complained that,

The fascination was in, 'Oh, where have you been; it's so bad, you poor thing', but there would be very little interest in how I got out of that hole and how I became well . . . Hugely interested in, 'Wow, you were in a coma for a few weeks, how terrible and suicidal and you've been locked up in psychiatric units for a few years of your life and it must be terrible' . . . Yes, it is. OK.

And then, well, the real interest should then be, 'How have you rebuilt your life? How have you got back into mainstream society, drive a car, get a job, get a girlfriend, have a house and not ended up completely on the scrapheap?'

Solution Focused Practitioners avoid giving advice, but peers will share their experiences of what works at Take Off (rather than reinforcing the illness with 'me too'). Mark noted,

In the early 2000s, when I was ill for the first time, I was suicidally depressed and I was a voluntary patient for the first time. There was literally nobody around who could say to me, 'I've done that, I've been there, I know what you're feeling, this is a helpful thing you might like to try'.

Within the Solution Focused therapy world, there is an ethos that the client is the expert in their own lives. One of the hardest things for professionals to learn when training in Solution Focused Practice (SFP) is to trust this to be true. However, this radical perspective is at the heart of the method, which uses questions to focus a person back onto their own strengths, resources, skills and preferences. The questions should help to 'stretch' a person's world of possibilities, encouraging them to think more broadly and creatively towards achieving a more satisfactory life and lifestyle (McKergow, 2021). One of the most reported benefits of using a Solution Focused approach for practitioners is a realisation (through practical experience) that the responsibility for change *can be* transferred to the client, that the client can be trusted to be an expert in their own life and to take positive steps towards creating a better future. This is different to some mental health training, which encourages practitioners to 'get the client to take responsibility', but lacks the question technology of SFP, and therefore often results in a feeling of failure or a projection of blame onto the client if they don't change.

As Take Off grew in the scope of its provision, new groups were set up and others retired through a process of trial and error. Any member could propose a group and, if they could gain enough interest, be funded to lead it. This model means that the groups offered by Take Off are always responsive to the members' needs and interests rather than determined by professionals. It has led to some imaginative and unique groups being set up, ranging from bicycle maintenance, beach cleans and online gaming groups. Take Off is securely funded in part by the local Mental Health Commissioner, who can see that Take Off is helping clients in a way that other organisations can't; they can see the improvement in the clients' behaviour, demeanour, attitude and outlook because the clients are learning from other people within the organisation. Take Off now attracts people from the age of 16, and the oldest person who comes is 86. As Mark Kilbey says:

Members represent every gender, every age and every type of background; an incredible diversity of people who come to Take Off and get something out of it because the defining, common similarity between people is experiencing the nightmares that your life can be, the destructiveness of mental ill health. So, you come through that door and I would like to think that people will automatically feel that they are safe. We had a lot of Asian members and fewer Black people. We were aware that some people faced particular discrimination in accessing services, but to be honest, we all faced difficulty accessing services, so it was always just about mutual support in Take Off.

The boldest group proposal was for a Peer Support Crisis Group for people in crisis or experiencing suicidal ideation. Mark describes the rationale:

We felt that the crisis services were becoming harder and harder to access; people were becoming more acutely ill before they were receiving any service at all. Because the funding for this group was limited, we wanted to look at the time of most need and we felt that, probably, the time when people were at most risk of self-harm or suicide, the time that they would probably find very little else available to them, would be a Sunday evening. And again, that was based on all our own experience.

Building on the existing success and working with the local Mental Health Commissioner, the group was set up and has been running successfully since 2015.

Unlike all the other groups at Take Off, the Peer Support Crisis Group (PSCG) is a referral-only group, requiring a referral from a GP, psychiatrist or Care Coordinator (sometimes called Lead Practitioner in other NHS Trusts). The group is funded by the local Integrated Care Board and provides a parallel service to the professional-led Kent and Medway NHS and Social Care Partnership Trust Crisis Teams, which can visit people in crisis at home. The group operates every Sunday between 4–8pm, 52 Sundays a year, which means it is also available during holidays such as Christmas and New Year. Three peer facilitators, trained in Solution Focused conversation, run the groups and up to 10 people attend each week. The group moved online during the COVID pandemic (and subsequent lockdowns) in the UK.

While the main activity in the group tends to be talking and socialising, there are also opportunities to engage in some activities like playing board games or food preparation.

In 2018, a year-long evaluation of the group was carried out. During this period, attendees were asked to complete a questionnaire at each attendance that covered the following elements:

- If you hadn't attended, what would you be doing instead?
- What difference has attending made to you?
- What did you like about attending today?
- What did you dislike?
- How comfortable did you feel?

At the end of the year, the data from 52 weeks was collected and analysed. To provide a richer insight into the experience of attending the PSCG, interviews were carried out with five attendees in February 2019 and with three PSCG facilitators in May 2019.

Out of 218 attendances (by 28 people in the year), 80% of these were considered 'useful' or 'very useful' and 99% of the time, people felt 'at ease' in the group. The data suggested that a 'usual Sunday evening' would be one where the person might be alone, isolated, lonely, bored or unoccupied by any meaningful activity, miserable or a more serious level of emotional distress, and at risk of self-harm or troublemaking. In contrast, the PSCG was reported to provide a space where people can be with others, socialise, have fun, be in a different location than home, engage in productive activities, experience emotional wellbeing and feel protected from risky behaviours. As one attendee stated, 'It can be a lifeline; it can be the difference between attending work for five days or having a complete breakdown'.

Attendees viewed the PSCG as a positive alternative to medical intervention. Some believed that if peer support had been available earlier in their psychiatric 'career', they might have required less medical intervention or developed greater coping skills earlier. One person said that going to Take Off, although very difficult, was preferable to having the Crisis Team (statutory service) visit because they didn't want people in their home. The sense of having 'somewhere to go' was echoed by other attendees.

> It just gives you somewhere to go to feel normal because everyone around you has got mental health issues; you feel better because you know they actually understand where you're coming from rather than talking to a counsellor, who's had training but doesn't actually get it.

The peer support workers and attendees are not necessarily aware of the significance of using Solution Focused Practice or how SFP compares to other therapeutic approaches. The training is light touch, and participants tend to use it because they quickly see the benefits – the questions are ones that they like to be asked and they have experienced personally that they feel better when talking about what they are doing, their strengths and preferred outcomes. This doesn't mean that people don't talk about their problems or what is currently bothering them.

For example, many shared that an important benefit of attendance was that they could share their thoughts and feelings without shocking or distressing others. They felt that friends' and family members' responses were often an additional source of stress or distress, which left them feeling isolated (because they felt they had to hide their thoughts and/or feelings), rejected or subject to scrutiny (because of others' fear).

> If I talk to friends, they kind of panic. But even with mental health professionals, their go-to answer is maybe you should be in hospital really and that's not always the case. It's just that possibly you just need someone to talk to.

However, their answers suggest that the crisis group facilitators were also moving conversations towards exceptions:

> It was really important for me to see that actually it [mental distress] is not necessarily something that has to be hidden and that there are lots of people who can speak about it **and** that there are people talking about living and working and not just about their difficulties.

It's in comments like this where we can see Solution Focused questions encouraging people to talk about what they are already doing and, characteristic of SFP's spotlight on 'exceptions', the times when the problem isn't happening or isn't so overwhelming (de Shazer, 1988).

Another comment suggests that the PSCG helps to create and then reinforce these instances:

> At some points during the group I still felt that depression, but there were points when I was distracted just by people's laughter and playing games and just watching.

Another element characteristic of SFP is being able to hold 'both/and', which is a good way to shift rigid thinking. We can see that in this comment: 'I think it just takes you out of your own head and almost forgetting that you're unwell because you're in a group of people who are unwell, but that doesn't seem to matter'.

Attendees felt that peers understood some of the paradoxes of mental illness whereby a person can be apparently functioning but also experiencing symptoms. This, they felt, was 'not permissible' when talking to mental health professionals who they thought would judge them as faking symptoms and withdraw support.

> You're living with the mental distress and, at the same time, you're living your life and it's like people don't want to let you do the two at the same time . . . I've said to them before, are you telling me that all the people who commit suicide weren't in employment?

The person went on to say,

> It's a shame they aren't asking me, 'How do you manage to be so resilient when you're also living with a mental illness?' That would be a more interesting question. It would be nice to be given some credit for doing that.

One more frequent user of the crisis group said that coming to Take Off had helped free them to 'be human, be able to do normal things'.

> I think I feel very bitter that I've had to put a hold on things that I've wanted to do in my life because of my mental health and because I'm not sitting there [at

home] ruminating; I'm not engaging in my very negative sort of behaviour such as self-harming. **It makes me feel like I can do something**.

They could see the value of the small achievements, which SFP helps people to connect to:

> I'm so disabled when I'm unwell; I cannot do anything, I can't think, I can't read, I can't sleep, I can't cook, I can't clean, I can't do anything and to be able to do a small thing like a human interaction, for me, that's a really big [achievement] . . . it's managing your goals and for me, if one of my goals was coming here and having a chat with a few people, well then that's the best thing that I'll do that day and that's actually ok.

This is an important point, and one that highlights the way that Solution Focused Practice helps to break overwhelming experiences by identifying and amplifying the exceptions to people's difficulties. It is important to hear this being described as a re-humanising experience.

While most of the benefits derived focus on what the individuals have gained personally from the groups, participants also perceive the benefit of being able to help others. This is the essence of peer support and while the facilitators are trained to run the group, the attendees also become aware that they can help each other. This can be by listening or offering strategies based on their own lived experiences. Following on from this realisation, some of the interviewees shared that they are now beginning to run other groups at Take Off and considering training as a Crisis Group facilitator. This could be explained by Grant and Gerrard's (2019) finding that using Solution Focused Practice increases self-efficacy and goal-setting.

Solution Focused practitioners do not need to be an 'expert' in other people and it is perhaps for this reason that peers are so comfortable using SFP and require less time to train. They do not need to unlearn previous knowledge. As Aine Garvey will explain later in this book, the approach has also been shown to cause much less stress to practitioners and reduce the risk of burnout. Through using SFP, practitioners will often report benefits in their own lives, as you don't need to be unwell or pathologised to find it useful. As one attendee said,

> When you help someone, by helping someone else with their problems, you're helping yourself; it doesn't make you feel better, it makes you feel like I've helped someone, I've made someone else's life better. And it spurs you on to try to help yourself, so it's like you help someone else, you help yourself, you sort of get a bit of both.

The insights from peers using and experiencing Solution Focused techniques could be useful to professionals working with those in mental health crisis, especially those already using Solution Focused approaches. Additionally, the success of the Take Off Peer Support Crisis Group suggests that Solution Focused conversation is a useful tool for peers to learn, as it brings together the deep empathy that is possible through shared experience with a set of simple questions (to explore and expand upon the small, too-oft overlooked instances of people's resourcefulness, skill and resilience).

When you talk to peers who are using and experiencing Solution Focused conversations, it becomes clear that they possess a particular knowledge about timing: how to balance talking about difficulties and solutions and a clarity of focus on exceptions. These service users are already experts by experience, and their training in the use of Solution Focused questions has enabled them to develop a unique, inclusive, peer-led support group, which helps themselves and others, at critical moments, to identify the strengths and qualities which can move them beyond the immediate crisis and towards safety and hope.

Note

1 Mental Health Charity Kent | Take Off | Canterbury.

References

de Shazer, S. (1988). *Clues: Investigating solutions in brief therapy*. W W Norton & Co.

Grant, A. M., & Gerrard, B. (2019). Comparing problem-focused, solution-focused and combined problem-focused/solution-focused coaching approach: solution-focused coaching questions mitigate the negative impact of dysfunctional attitudes. *Coaching: An International Journal of Theory, Research and Practice, 13*(1), 61–77. https://doi.org/10.1080/17521882.2019.1599030.

McKergow, M. (2021). *The next generation of solution focused practice: Stretching the world for new opportunities and progress*. Routledge.

Shalaby, R., & Agyapong, V. (2020). Peer support in mental health: Literature review. *JMIR Mental Health, 7*(6). https://doi.org/10.2196/15572.

Chapter 8

Using Solution Focused Practice to shape mental health services for children and young people

Natasha Adams

I really think that the focus on solution-finding with young people can make a huge difference. It's such an important part of their journey, yet it seems to be one of the things that are often overlooked in care plans, preferring a focus on fixing the young person's response – rather than a dual focus on response and environment.

This is Claire Hartshorn, CYPS Transformation Manager, Surrey Child & Adolescent Mental Health Services (CAMHS), in a discussion between the two of us in August 2024. The conversation consolidated our shared learning following a pilot project with Surrey Community CAMHS service for young people on a long waiting list for support. The conversation reflected upon and discussed the benefits of using SFP as a waiting-well and whole CAMHS toolkit for young people presenting with self-harm and/or suicidal ideation.

Learning Space

Learning Space is a Solution Focused children and young person's mental health charity which sees children as young as 5 and up to age 18 and works closely with parents and carers.

Practitioners and mentors make up a multi-disciplinary team with backgrounds in social work, art and drama therapy, counselling, youth work, teaching and early years, autism and ADHD specialisms.

The charity's relationship with BRIEF (www.brief.org.uk) started in 1997; and BRIEF has been the provider of practitioner and mentor training as part of staff induction within the charity.

I remember my excitement at attending BRIEF's training where I was among participants from around the world in the fields of educational psychology and social work.

The discovery that Solution Focused Practice (SFP) involves a not-knowing approach, that clients' 'best hopes' can be located within everyday lives, that clients are treated as the expert and that SFP can work very well with little – if any – historical information, was mind-blowing.

DOI: 10.4324/9781003519225-8

I was excited at the prospect of bringing together SFP and youth work. With a wonderful team of creative mentors and young people sharing their ideas of accessible services, 121SPACE was created – a blend of community-placed 1:1 groups and activities, a project spanning five years, supporting hundreds of young people in a way that was right for them; their best hopes being central to the support (as part of Learning Space's Early Help Commission with Surrey County Council).

And the creation of 121SPACE was just the beginning.

A Solution Focused approach across systems

The success of developing and implementing a child and young person-led Solution Focused Triage within Surrey's Mindworks (new CAMHS) access and advice service has had ripples – creating curiosity, interest and further opportunities to simplify systems. Over time, we have begun to grow a dynamic culture of shared learning, cutting through organisational challenges and complex systems and privileging young people's voices through Solution Focused approaches.

In partnership with East Surrey Place primary care networks, we have co-created Young Person Link Worker roles, integrating Solution Focused Practice to promote the voice of families early so that families are treated as the experts in their own lives.

These roles will model a system wide strength-based, Solution Focused approach which listens to families when they need help. This is in response to an identified problem where children, young people and families face a lot of confusion over what emotional wellbeing and mental health services are available, how to access them and what services would be most beneficial to them. This results in families bouncing around a complex system.

The ambition is to bring together services to co-produce and model a place-based offer which can support client autonomy and accessibility in a safe and timely manner. Key to this work will be a Solution Focused Triage model, operating within the THRIVE framework which will celebrate family strengths, as well highlight system need.[1]

How did it all start?

In 2021, Mindsight Child & Adolescent Mental Health Services (CAMHS) went through a major transformation. Learning Space became one of 13 charities making up the new Surrey CAMHS, together with SABP (Surrey and Borders Partnership NHS Trust) and the Tavistock and Portman Thrive Framework for system change:

We know that existing provision of Children's Emotional Wellbeing & Mental Health services in Surrey does not always meet the standards that we expect and that our children and young people deserve.

Some children and young people can wait longer than they should before they receive assessment and treatment. There are unacceptable delays for children and young people in need of support.

Existing service provision, based on a traditional model of assessment and treatment is limiting for some children and young people and does not fully respond to their needs.[2]

Learning Space Mindworks offers community wellbeing services, 1:1 and ND (neurodivergent-specific) services for children and young people with or without a diagnoses of autism and or ADHD (Attention Deficit Hyperactivity Disorder).

The aim of the new service was to make children and young people's voices central to their care by offering a mix of clinical and non-clinical interventions.[3]

The THRIVE Framework

The Tavistock and Portman THRIVE framework[4] sat central to the new system, ensuring that services provided:

- Shared decision-making – *the process is as important as the outcome* – and give families a good experience of having their wishes heard
- Accessibility to timely advice, help and risk support in local communities – where children, young people and their families are – and in a way that best suits them
- Proactive prevention and promotion – to enable the whole community to support mental health and wellbeing
- Outcome-informed interventions with clear and transparent goals, measures of progress and action plans

Young people and parent/carer's best hopes for the new service

In 2021, before the launch of the new Mindworks service, Learning Space led several events for young people and families giving the system an opportunity to hear clients' best hopes for a service that would meet a child and young person's needs in a way, and at the time, they needed help.

Children, young people and their families identified that they wanted greater involvement in the decisions made about their care, a quicker and smoother process to access services and transition between services, and a stronger focus on positive attributes within the family to build their confidence and sense of self-worth.

'Services need to not only focus on the problems but also the young people's successes and make them feel valued and secure as they feel they can share the good, the bad and the difficulties', was one young person's feedback.

A parent wrote:

> I'm the parent of a 14-year-old just diagnosed with autism. We've been in and out of the CAMHS system for around seven years with no support and the diagnosis pathway took over two years. Now we have the diagnosis, but we feel like we're left hanging as no follow-up was offered, so the reasons for the initial referral are left unaddressed. The service needs to be speedy and holistic – to have a child tell you that they want help but know that they are not bad enough for CAMHS to take seriously is heartbreaking.

Another said:

> I hope the new service will be fully committed to working in respectful partnership with parents, listening to them as regards to their child's difficulties and what [help] they might need to 'engage', keeping in touch and taking concerns seriously. Many parents have been 'blamed', laughed at, patronised, contradicted in front of their distressed children and their extensive experience of their child's troubles ignored, to the detriment of the child.

Place-based services

Community Wellbeing Services were geographically split between six charities. Learning Space covers three areas:

- Mole Valley
- Reigate and Banstead
- Epsom and Ewell

Building on the success of the Early Help model, we embraced what was working well and co-created our Community Wellbeing place-based offer based on what children, young people, parents, schools, services and practitioners were telling us.
    We did this by:

- Listening to what children, young people and parents were telling us, with their best hopes as a starting point
- Being proactive in understanding the emerging needs and access barriers
- Working within the THRIVE framework
- Solution Focused Practice being central to all discussions

Our menu included:

- Parent empowerment courses – online and in-person
- Forest Space and creative groups for children not accessing education
- Community placed one-to-one support; coffee shops, walk in the park, in-school sessions

- School-based transition groups
- Social groups for children and young people experiencing high levels of anxiety, using indoor and outdoor spaces
- Advocacy groups for young people and parents/carers; a space for young people and parents to inform service change, celebrate what's working well and say what could be different. Raising LGBTQI awareness and neurodivergence awareness in schools

A Solution Focused Triage – Phase One

A year into the contract, the service was significantly over-subscribed, with an increase in requests for support for younger children and the presentation of more complex mental health needs.

Through our work, we noticed that when a child or young person comes into the system, families often receive a problem-focused contact inviting detailed questions about the problem – 'How long have you been experiencing the problem?', 'When did the problems start?'. We also noticed that children's and young people's voices were not being routinely recorded and that professionals in the system were the experts, making decisions as to what service would be best for the child and young person.

Learning Space met with the access and advice team to discuss a new way of triaging families at the point of referral. We proposed a Solution Focused Triage pilot for families living in our Community Wellbeing areas.

A total of 18 children, young people and families from East Surrey took part in the pilot in May 2022. The families were from East Surrey, which covered our Community Wellbeing offer.

Eighteen referrals were received and accepted from access and advice for children aged 7 to 15 years old.

How did we go about the Triage?

Our own best hope was to construct a placed-based Solution Focused Triage model offering choice and genuine shared decision-making with the child's and young person's voice front and centre. Our place-based menu and knowledge of local services would support this.

The Triage team worked closely with our community wellbeing administrator to ensure we could ensure families would be seen within a two-week period and that, as a system, we were working to the child's (and family's) best hope as recorded. The child and young person's voice was paramount and was our priority.

We offered in-person or online meetings and could offer outreach for families unable to access either. The Triage was offered to children and young people, inclusive of autism, ADHD or being neurotypical.

We introduced a Solution Focused script to ensure we kept close to the intentions of the Triage. It was important for us to assume the Triage could be an intervention in itself – this might be enough for families.

We wanted to experiment with the approach to ensure we created a safe space that reduced fear and anxiety as quickly as possible, giving the best opportunity to feel and be safe, maybe even to have fun and provide some control over choices. We wanted to amplify strengths and resources with the intention that families felt safe when they walked out of the room.

And we did!

Triage pilot – outcomes and learning

The evidence from the Triage pilot showed that clients were co-creating their own support regardless of how they came into the service and perhaps challenged not only the wider organisational system but also their own. I was particularly surprised that 75% of young people who had or were awaiting a diagnosis of autism felt their immediate needs (building confidence, family relations and coping mechanisms) could be met within the community well-being or parent anxiety group and did not feel an automatic referral to the neuro-developmental team was needed.

This is what we learnt from the data:

- Children and young people were seen within a two-week period
- 18% didn't require a service as family strengths were elevated and found they could cope without support
- The Triage enabled parents to identify changes needed in school – access to a time-out card, for example, SEN assessments, access to support in school
- The Triage drew on family strengths to cope, celebrating what was working well
- Triage intervention identified when to escalate to crisis services and supported safety planning

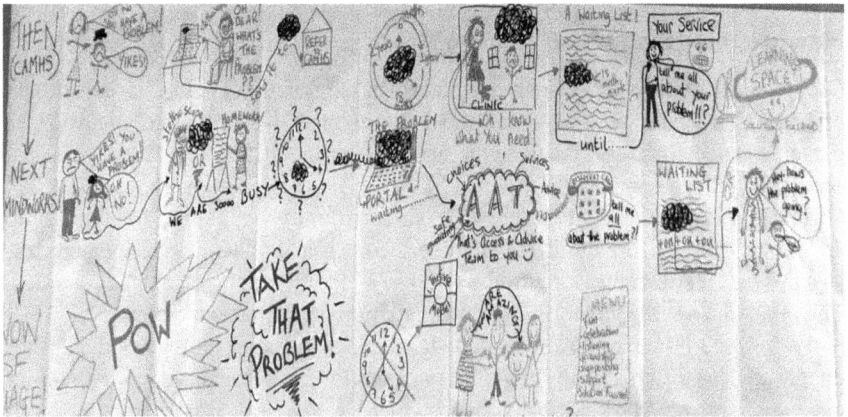

Figure 8.1 Sarah Charlton, senior community mentor for Learning Space, uses her creative expertise to illustrate the introduction of Solution Focused Practice as a catalyst for change within complex mental health systems, telling the story of the pilot.

- 41% chose a six-session 1:1 SF support service
- 19% opted for a community based 1:1 offer
- 22% opted for a group

Risk assessments in real-time

Although pilot referrals were screened for any safeguarding concerns, we discovered 'best hopes conversations' invited client disclosures of self-harm, suicidal ideation and family breakdown. The early co-constructed intervention meant safety plans could be created in that moment, and further support needs could be identified, all the while staying Solution Focused and keeping the clients' best hopes at the very centre of things: fitting with their reality and placing them in a position of control of their own and the wider system of support.

Practitioner learning and motivation

Imperative to growing the Solution Focused Triage culture were weekly practitioner meetings which focused on:

- Case study discussions
- Presentation of work that we were pleased with or surprised to notice
- What were we learning from children, young people and families – asking, 'How can we do more of this?'
- Discovering our stylistic approaches to having useful conversations – capturing the voices of neuro-divergent clients; use of kinaesthetic scaling and whole family discussions

We were energised, inspired and motivated by the success of this approach and the co-constructed aesthetic we were privileged to be a part of. Seeing children (as young as 6), young people and families challenging the assumptions and expectations set within their own systems and being the catalyst for change was a very powerful experience for us. Aine Garvey will look in more detail about the impact of SFP on practitioner wellbeing later in this book.

I discovered that inviting 'When are you at your best?' conversations at the very beginning gave space for children, young people and families to be celebrated and seen outside of the problem – enabling strengths and celebrated qualities to be woven throughout the Triage.

The pilot was seen as a success and subsequently written up as a THRIVE 'getting advice and signposting implementation story'.[5]

Solution Focused Triage – Phase Two

With the success of the pilot, Learning Space felt well-placed to offer self-referral routes to families needing help. The pilot provided the potential for whole system change, both in the context of families and mental health services. The Triage model also provided a framework to meet families when they needed help: building a culture of inclusivity, safety and hope.

Integrating Solution Focused Practice throughout the organisation

Keen to consolidate the success of the Triage (I was mindful that this could easily become diluted due to contractual requirements and service demand), and with administrators being families' first point of contact, it felt important to give our administrators an experience of SFP as well. This came in the form of in-house training and peer supervision.

Case Study 1

Mum (Summer) felt online would be the best way of capturing her son Max's voice. She didn't think he would speak to me, but we agreed to give it a try. I knew that Max had experienced a number of crises, suicide attempts, some domestic abuse, drug use and physical bullying. I knew that Max was on a long waiting list for support from a young people's clinician.

Sticking with my SF script, starting with 'at your best', Max proceeded to reel off a long list of survival techniques and proud to notice examples that had kept him safe, stimulated and hopeful for his future. Max was animated and enthusiastic to share his IT talents and special interests, and together, Summer and Max celebrated their journeys in understanding their ADHD and Autism, finding a language to communicate and respond to safety needs, celebrating their resilience and being unapologetically themselves. I offered two further sessions, which were not taken up and both felt they had the resources to cope moving forwards.

Between November 2022 and 2024, Learning Space triaged a further 300 families. Children aged 6 to 18 years old were invited to face-to-face triage meetings. A small percentage opted for online sessions as this was the safest and most practical means of accessing the space. Our place-based menu provided choices for children, young people and families. Children opted for groups instead of long-term 1:1 support and associated these with 'being happy', 'more confident', 'feeling accepted'. Menus were offered to parents, freeing the child from being the focus of family difficulties.

Risk assessment in real-time

'At my best' and 'best hopes' questions formed the basis of support conversations (verbal and non-verbal) with children and young people around safety and risk and invited discussions around the reality of staying alive, being able to cope, being brave enough to attend the session and so on, leading to the co-creation of safety plans.

This approach worked extremely well with families, too.

Case Study 2

A triage session with an 11-year-old and her mother identified that mum's battle with cancer and their eldest son's physical and emotional reaction to it had contributed to family breakdown.

The daughter wanted her brother to be kind to her, and the mother wanted the family to get on together like they used to. The Triage gave a space to hear the importance of their cultural identity and beautiful descriptions of their Arabic names, celebrating when times were good and describing courage, love and hope.

The outcome of the Triage was that the family would have a Solution Focused family session together.

Mum, dad, older brother (16), younger sister (11) and younger brother (9) attended, positioning themselves in a circle. The youngest child was excited to take the role of note-taker and did an expert job of capturing individual and family strengths, best hopes and 'exceptions'. Family members proudly shared their Arabic names and meanings – adding personal stories to the translations. Their 'best hopes' (to spend more time together) created a supportive atmosphere, allowing for descriptions of love, bravery, survival and thoughts about the future.

Dad shared his joy of the moments within the preferred future amidst the chaos of his reality, of being a witness to his beautiful family, who he so clearly adored.

The eldest son shared his awareness of the impact he had on the family and his wish to move forwards and to go back to college, to understand his ADHD better and to feel accepted.

Mum watched with pride, giving centre-stage to her husband and children, enjoying the laughter and love so evidently in front of her.

I suggested that when they went about their day-to-day life, they imagined doing some 'invisible fishing', sharing the idea that they might try and catch moments they were pleased with or surprised to notice.

I followed up with Mum the following week. With excitement, she listed what she described as 'mini miracles' following the session. The elder brother had been to see his younger sister perform at gymnastics; they had all been out for a dog walk together; dad had got all the children ready for school and brought breakfast in bed for mum; and mum was setting aside some time for herself to think about returning to teaching.

Mum's final words were that 'we each have the love and power to get through anything' and 'it was beautiful to see my family's love, gratitude and appreciation for one another despite the challenges we have been through'.

Conclusion

The success and impact of the Solution Focused Triage have generated curiosity and interest across systems, including Mindworks and Primary Care Networks (PCN's), both of which are funded by the NHS. Since September 2023, Learning Space has hosted two full-time PCN posts with Dorking Healthcare and Redhill Phoenix, working closely with GP practices. The Solution Focused Triage sits central to this and provides an easier route for families to access help, allowing GPs to focus on patient care and spend less time making referrals.

Learning Space has piloted Waiting Well services in response to rising levels of need and complexities in the Mindworks system: these services provide a safe space for children and young people to co-create alternative routes to safety and hope. Surrey is seeing a growing social model approach to health and wellbeing, and with Learning Space's growing involvement within the Primary Care Network, we can make sure that SFP continues to inspire hope, cultural celebration, resilience and choice.

Although the Learning Space journey using a Solution Focused Triage model is just one small placed-based example of how SFP can impact clinical systems, it is doing so. Gradually, we are removing some of the pressures placed on specialist neurodivergent services and GPs, who were previously the only solutions, and we are beginning to present a strong case to grow a social model of care in our area.

Society – including our Health and Social Care systems – has conditioned us to think in problem-focused ways. Therefore, the task of implementing a Solution Focused Triage across complex mental health systems (whether this be for children and adolescents, working-age adults or older adults) requires mindful and deliberate changes to the process to avoid practitioners slipping into a familiar 'fixing and knowing best' mode.

Where we manage to achieve this, reflective space for practitioners to celebrate what they have been pleased with or surprised to notice in their work – holding firm to a belief and trust in clients of all ages – helps to create clinical environments that can celebrate family capability, diversity and culture; and will help to provide the inclusivity, safety and hope required for the ownership of support plans and the overcoming of crises towards lives containing best hopes.

My own best hope is that this book will contribute to the change that will be necessary within organisations to embrace Solution Focused Practice as a simple, yet radical approach to instilling respect and celebrating the capabilities of individuals and families.

What might this look like?

Let's imagine that when you wake up tomorrow, you have the opportunity to see each person you talk to as they really are – without assumptions, without an agenda, without conditions or any diagnosis you might be aware of. To see them and to hear them, however they need to communicate, having the absolute privilege of facilitating and observing their creative process and truly celebrating their cultural identity. And suppose you helped to collect a list of their strengths and to hear these spoken out loud. What difference might this start to make?

If you are interested in watching the ripples of SF possibility in your own organisation, I'd be very happy to connect. Please email me at: sfnatasha.adams@gmail.com.

Notes

1   Taken from the Young Person Link Worker job description, Adams, N., & Turner, L. (2024, July). *Senior programme manager for prevention and communities*. Surrey Heartlands NHS Foundation Trust. www.eastsurrey-alliance.org/children-and-young-peoples-services

2   Shared at user voice engagement event, co-facilitated by Learning Space. Written up in a Briefing for Parents, produced by Surrey Children's Emotional Wellbeing & Mental Health Services.

3   www.mindworks-surrey.org/our-services/neurodevelopmental-services/learning-space

4   THRIVE Framework for system change | i-THRIVE

5   https://implementingthrive.org/implemented/case-studies-2/getting-advice-and-signposting-case-studies/

Chapter 9

Statutory Children's workers

'Modelling hope' to engage and support young people in crisis

Luke Goldie-McSorley

Models and modelling come up a lot when talking or thinking about children and young people. And there are two meanings for the purposes of this chapter: 'What model will you be using?' and also 'You might be a good role model for them'/'They could do with a solid role model'.

I have been labelled like this – acceptingly and begrudgingly – throughout my career. I have also often spoken about a model I rely upon in my interventions with young people: Solution Focused Practice.

In this chapter, I will explain my theory of Solution Focused Practice with young people in crisis and how Solution Focused Practice is, in my view, the ultimate co-conspirator to modelling hope and 'being the hope' when working, talking to and *being* with young people in crisis.

I am now 11 years qualified as a social worker: working within services for children and adolescents, first of all within frontline and 'Edge of Care' local authority social work, and now in Child and Adolescent Mental Health Services (CAMHS). I reflect on this time and journey and think about my determination and drive to practice with people: to intervene therapeutically in a purposeful and connected way, filled with hope. Maybe I have become a 'hope model' as much as a role model.

Hope is the expectation and/or desire for positive events or moments in the future (Hayes et al., 2017) and Snyder et al. (1997) describe hope as the ability to see the route to your goals as well as bringing forth the agency needed to take those routes to achieve the said goals. In situations of crisis, many of our thoughts or typical structures of practice can be set aside whilst we 'deal with the crisis'. I argue that hope in those early moments can be experienced as healing, a basis from which to build towards goal achievement (Idris et al., 2023) and the beginnings of recovery: a route out of the crisis.

Whilst I don't love the term 'direct work', I do love working directly with young people, training others and growing my experience in using Solution Focused Practice with my clients. My Solution Focused Practice has been delivered in a variety of settings, situations and contexts: from fields, to homes, to placements, to clinic settings, to phone calls, to smartphone chats and more.

DOI: 10.4324/9781003519225-9

I have taken part in a whole range of satisfying conversations: those beginning conversations when we first meet, the one-off conversations, the long-standing relationship conversations, the therapy, the maintenance, the endings and the crisis. It is the crisis conversations that I will focus on within this chapter: the different forms these take and how Solution Focused Practice (SFP) embodies, develops and invites hope in those we talk with who are in crisis.

I want to celebrate the power of hope and show how it is used in SFP. As I write, rates of probable mental disorders in children and young people remain at one in five (NHS England, 2023) and self-injurious behaviours are one of the leading causes of death globally in young people (Jerome et al., 2024). There is great pressure and stress on children and young people as well as services to support them. Hope is a protective factor against suicide risk in adolescents (Pharris et al., 2023), and SFP can be one route to establishing that.

All the transcripts and examples I have provided in this chapter have been anonymised to protect the confidentiality of the clients or a combination of clients whose stories I will use.

How I use Solution Focused Practice with children and young people

When starting to work with a young person, I realise that I always ask, 'What are your best hopes?' or find an alternative way to invite a young person to think about a desired outcome for their life or from treatment. This question alone can have a huge impact on young people (even when asked by practitioners who are just beginning to learn the approach). The describing of an outcome, for example, the slightest reduction in distress or greater happiness, is a future-focused cognitive process. Pharris et al. (2023) state that hope is also a future-focused cognitive process that can be nurtured and consistently contributes to resilience in the face of difficulty or crisis. I would argue that 'hope nurturing' is a key aspect of inviting someone to describe a desired outcome for their life or moments where they have already experienced the outcome they want for themselves.

In one situation where I had just met a young person who had such lengthy experiences of challenge, trauma and crisis that they felt hope and future change wasn't for them – that it just wasn't possible – I recall the power (in the first session) of simply asking the question 'What are your hopes from this?'. There were moments where I needed to re-phrase the question, offer long pauses and wait patiently so the essence of the question could be thoroughly absorbed. In this instance, the young person answered that they would 'understand themselves'. I asked what difference this would make to them, and they found it difficult to tell me the answer straight away.

As Evan George has described in his chapter, the beauty of this approach is its belief and hope in what Solution Focused questions can do and what the young person themselves can do with the questions. As our talking progressed through topics they wished to share and instances where life had been really hard, as well as momentarily successful, the belief in the best hopes question and in their own answer never left the room. This culminated in arriving back at the difference it might make to them, and the way we had journeyed around in the meantime enabled the young person to say they 'would feel control and freedom in themselves'. This outcome was as far as our talking reached that day in terms of a structured SFP intervention; however, what became clear when we next met over a week later was that imagined differences had already begun to take hold, changes they felt they could make in their life and power they felt beginning to grow in themselves. All from a desired outcome conversation.

Tips that might be useful in practice

I find that holding onto a desired outcome or inviting an outcome shifts some of the stuckness or worry of crisis. Doing so allows for the fact that there are multiple routes to that outcome, many of which we could not devise or come up with as practitioners, so allowing room for those to come through can only be helpful. Ask the best hopes or desired outcome question in all contexts, even if you can't ask anything else, and expect the routes to that outcome to be hugely varied and unexpected.

In many ways, the simplest tip to provide is to listen. Listen in a way that creates a bubble around you and the client (Perry & Goldie-McSorley, 2024). I have often described my sessions as feeling like the development of a bubble which will contain and grow hope and which will acknowledge difficulty and struggle, as well as progress, difference and success. Time after time, the feedback from young people is about the listening: they felt I had allowed them room to think and grow and try. So listen – so hard that you only hear their words.

An approach to practice and a practice model

Over time, through hours and hours of practice with hundreds of clients, as well as many hours of delivering SFP training, I've become fond of and connected to describing Solution Focused Practice as an 'Approach to Practice and a Practice Model'. The practice model is simply the structured conversational rules and techniques – not least the building of the next question from the client's answer. I see the *approach to practice* as my strong connection with hope and the modelling of that hope to young people. This is the stance from which we as Solution Focused practitioners view, hold in mind, think about, speak *to* and speak *about* the people we work with or support. It affects how we write about them and write to them.

Tips that might be useful in practice

The way in which we write to young people, in letters about treatment, formulations and assessments can directly impact a hopeful future, a route towards recovery. It is so vital we write as the version of ourselves we hope to be in the therapy room (and outside): to be tentative and caring, to look to invite helpful thoughts and to plant seeds with our words and messages.

SFP assumptions and genuine care

The SFP approach and assumptions are an all-encompassing way in which we care for people. Our stance includes the following:

1 People have their own good reasons for doing what they do
2 There is not necessarily a logical connection between the problem and the solution
3 Trusting the client allows them to be creative and change
4 No problem happens all the time, and no one is perfect at their problems; there are always exceptions/instances of success
5 Change is constant and inevitable
6 A small change can lead to bigger changes
7 People bring with them many resources and strengths
8 Nothing is pre-determined – the future can be created and is negotiable

I think about these assumptions as faders in my therapeutic mixer desk: varying points from which I will need to dial up or dial down.

When modelling hope for young people in crisis, I would regularly, internally, refer back to this list of assumptions, not to attempt to solve their crisis or their situation, but instead to create a basis from which I can develop my Solution Focused questions: to find the right structure for my clients and persist with seeking a conversation that fits well with them.

Tips that might be useful in practice

When working with young people experiencing mental health crises, my advice to other practitioners is to find means which allow you to slow down and think: to be the best workplace version of yourself. I fervently believe that the assumptions I have outlined previously are a means to slow down our practice, giving us time to think about the questions and interventions that will be asked and made by our best professional selves.

The absorption of these assumptions not only helps us to be the best version of ourselves for our clients but will give our clients the most useful experience and opportunity for recovery. Solution Focused Practice prioritises the agency, power and capability of the client. Trusting relationships filled with hope and belief are strongly linked to recovered mental health (Russinova, 1999). This involves a clear belief from practitioners regarding their clients' abilities to recover or succeed (Murphy et al., 2024).

What does the literature say?

When working with young people in mental health crises and thinking about hope, I believe we must take account of the literature on recovery.

For those experiencing mental disorders, hope is an integral factor of recovery (Ellison et al., 2018) and many models of recovery stress that hope is a critical aspect of persons being able to live a satisfactory life undefined by their illness (Hayes et al., 2017). Barber (2012) writes about recovery in three ways, though these are not mutually exclusive: the cure or remission of symptoms, symptom control and personal recovery. This aligns with Anthony's (1993) notion of recovery, in which a person acknowledges their illness whilst not being defined by it and continues to strive, with hope, for a life worth having.

The SFP assumptions that I have referred to invite a position of not knowing (Flatt & Curtis, 2013) and an acceptance of uncertainty. Embodying SFP allows me as a practitioner to sit comfortably with the uncertainty of outcomes, as my focus relies upon and remains guided by my constant belief in the client's outcome happening. Even when measures or restrictions must be put in place for safety reasons, this belief does not diminish.

Tips that might be useful in practice

Everything we do must communicate our hope: when we *are* in the room with young people and when we are *not*. Whilst we complete tasks, ask required questions, talk therapeutically, invite reflection and even complete questionnaires, we have to exude and communicate hope for the people who are seeing us: hope that a desired outcome is possible, that difference is around the corner and that recovery can be arrived at via varying routes.

Being content and comfortable with uncertainty is crucial. We can never know what's landing for young people. If I get signs something isn't working or useful, then I hold the responsibility to try and find another angle, a different jumping-off point or another way to fit with the client. What helps me to do that is hard listening, listening for the words or moments to hook a question on, with no clear plan or agenda – just a mindful aligning of the next step with what I am hearing from the young person.

Description of a future where the client's outcome is present, whatever that outcome may be, requires both trust and some form of imagination. A future that has not yet been determined or negotiated is a space where hope can be fostered – even in moments when people feel at their very worst. Hope combined with imagination allows for things to happen that may not have felt possible before (Murphy et al., 2024).

Having a plan but keeping it simple

I remember a phone call with a young person who was finding it harder and harder to cope with their mental health difficulty. We were able to slow down our conversation just enough to share a description of what a slight reduction in their symptoms (and the impact of this) would look like.

Through slow and purposeful use of SFP, I invited them to describe four small instances which might show them the difference that a reduction in symptoms would make. Within each instance, I was able to ask about the observable differences they would notice in themselves: what they would do, how they would do it and what others might notice? We discussed brief pre-suppositional interactions[1] with others and the differences a reduction of symptoms would make.

We were able to move around in timespan as the young person described the presence of differences in their future and then moved to lists of things, behaviours and thoughts that have helped before. This phone call became filled with detail that began to paint a picture of possibility and, of course, possibility brings hope.

My belief in the SFP process is shown through asking the questions and creating the time and space for the answers. It is shown by continuing to invite more detail based upon a previous answer, which was directly connected to the young person's hope for the reduction of their symptoms and distress. I was able to hear and dwell helpfully on many details which fitted with the version of that young person in a life with fewer symptoms, less distress and a consolidated recovery.

In my experience, the questions, stance and focus of the model create a connection, which in turn becomes a relationship – or alliance – from which positive difference and impactful intervention happens. This solidity is very useful in moments of crisis where the ground can feel as though it is giving way beneath the young people's feet, where the tightrope they feel they are on is swaying and previously reliable safety ropes are coming loose.

Hope isn't given by a helping professional or created by them: much like SFP, it relies on co-construction and trust (Goldie-McSorley in Yusuf, 2021). Solution Focused conversations don't start with a plan, especially in crisis situations. The key to the approach is that the next question is developed from the last answer; the practitioner and young person take turns speaking and the practitioner shows care and hard listening. Murphy et al. (2024) suggest hope is either uncovered where already present or is constructed between persons in a trusting and caring interaction, which in every sense aligns with Solution Focused Practice.

Here is a brief transcript of work with a young person in crisis. They were giving up, crowded by people; giving up on themselves and possibility:

The following interaction comes with me knelt on the floor with the young person.

Luke: Can I sit?
Client: *No answer, no look, no movement.*
Luke: I don't want to sit and be another person crowding you, and I just wondered whether we could talk just a little, in a good way for you?
Client: Nothing, there's nothing. I give up; I don't want to talk.
Luke: Ok, what if just us, *we* found something in our talking that might make just the slightest difference? Can we try?

At this moment, I can feel the bubble around us; nothing else really exists. All that is present is me, my colleague, the client, the content they provide, the Solution Focused Practice structure and language and hope, all in a closed bubble.

Client: *Shrugs but looks at us.*
Luke: *Putting my arm out.* We got you. Let's find a way together to talk that helps, or we can just sit and not talk, we got you . . .
Client: *Linked arms and walked together to seats.*

Tips that might be useful in practice

Reviewing and checking in with people is an opportunity to invite hope and difference. Whilst assessing the risks, we can assess the hope and invite some more. We can dial up our faders in those calls, sessions, meetings and interactions.

In the exchange mentioned previously, we made sure that progress was very slow. We asked the question (whilst acknowledging everything that came before): 'If this talking was helpful right now, what might it lead to?'. We described together some coping in the next hour, some signs that they were getting through, some signs of the tiniest glimmer of hope returning, and what they might hope to notice in the coming days before we visited again.

Total recovery can be overwhelming. Instead, focus on small parts of it. One way I do this is to hold in mind that much of my efforts are to keep the young person 'in the room' or in the conversation as long as possible. For as long as they are in the conversation, then, they are able to think and hear questions, have new thoughts and gather new insights. Without them being there, I can't be useful, so keep them in the room long enough for them to begin to think.

Practitioners must be modellers of hope, candles of hope or reservoirs of hope (Murphy et al., 2024). The hope in question is produced by effective use and belief in SFP and its values. It is something that is inherent in the structure of SFP and becomes part of practitioners themselves. As Aine Garvey writes later in this book, it is an important aspect of what keeps practitioners using the approach; it's what pushes against the tides and waves of burnout in statutory work with children and young people; it's what keeps us believing in what is possible, especially for those in crisis.

Conclusion

Working with young people who may not ordinarily access therapeutic support is a privilege – it's a precious moment in time to be grabbed with both hands. Whilst mental health crisis may be the precipitating factor, hope is the required mitigator. Working in services for children and young people might not always fill practitioners with hope, but when thinking about recovery and intervention and the differences short conversations can make, surely hope is vital and continuously an option. Modelling hope is my biggest tip to a practitioner looking to make a difference to a young person in crisis. Take the opportunity to ask some questions which evidence how hopeful you are for the person, their situation and their recovery. Hope and recovery are mates, and I argue that there is no better way to create hope in distressed young people than by asking Solution Focused questions. Go on, give it a try. I dare you!

Note

1 A presupposition is something that is assumed beforehand at the outset of a line of argument or course of action. In SFP, presuppositional interactions are commonplace (Froerer et al., 2023) and are interactions with the assumption that the other person is capable of success, change and action and they have past experience of skill, strength, capacity aligned to the hoped-for changes they desire.

References

Anthony, W. A. (1993). Recovery from mental illness: The guiding vision of the mental health service system in the 1990s. *Psychosocial Rehabilitation Journal, 16(4),* 11. https://doi.org/10.1037/h0095655.

Barber, M. E. (2012). Recovery as the new medical model for psychiatry. *Psychiatric Services, 63(3),* 277–279. https://doi.org/10.1176/appi.ps.201100248.

Ellison, M. L., Belanger, L. K., Niles, B. L., Evans, L. C. & Bauer, M. S. (2018). Explication and definition of mental health recovery: A systematic review. *Administration and Policy in Mental Health and Mental Health Services Research, 45*(1), 91–102. https://doi.org/10.1007/s10488-016-0767-9.

Flatt, S., & Curtis, S. (2013). Offering expert knowledge within a not-knowing solution-focused paradigm: A contradiction in terms or a helpful response to (some) real life conundrums. *International Journal of Solution-Focused Practices, 1(1)*, 28–30. https://doi.org/10.14335/ijsfp.v1i1.12.

Froerer, A. S., Walker, C. R., & Lange, P. (2023). Solution focused brief therapy presuppositions: A comparison of 1.0 and 2.0 SFBT approaches. *Contemporary Family Therapy, 45*, 425–436. https://doi.org/10.1007/s10591-022-09654-5.

Goldie-McSorley, L. (2021). Trusting the child: Using the solution focused approach with children and young people on the edge of care. In D. Yusuf (Ed.), *The solution focused approach with children and young people* (pp. 123–129). Routledge.

Hayes, L., Herrman, H., Castle, D., & Harvey, C. (2017). Hope, recovery and symptoms: The importance of hope for people living with severe mental illness. *Australasian Psychiatry: Bulletin of the Royal Australian and New Zealand College of Psychiatrists, 25*(6), 583–587. https://doi.org/10.1177/1039856217726693.

Idris, A., Akhir, N. M., Mohamad, M. S., & Sarnon, N. (2023). Exploring the lived experience on recovery from major depressive disorder (MDD) among women survivors and five CHIME concepts: A qualitative study. *Behavioral Sciences, 13*(2), 151. https://doi.org/10.3390/bs13020151.

Jerome, L., Masood, S., Henden, J., Bird, V., & Ougrin, D. (2024). Solution-focused approaches for treating self-injurious thoughts and behaviours: A scoping review. *BMC Psychiatry, 24*(1), 646. https://doi.org/10.1186/s12888-024-06101-7.

Murphy, J., Mulcahy, H., Mahony, J. O., Bradley, S., & Ryan, D. (2024). Exploring individuals' experiences of hope in mental health recovery: Having a sense of possibility. *Journal of Psychiatric and Mental Health Nursing, 31*(4), 617–627. https://doi.org/10.1111/jpm.13013.

NHS England. (2023). *Mental health of children and young people in England, 2023 – wave 4 follow up to the 2017 survey.* NHS England Digital.

Perry, N., & Goldie-McSorley, L. (2024). Suspending disbelief – Using solution focused practice with young people in mental health crisis. *Journal of Solution Focused Practices, 8*(2). https://doi.org/10.59874/001c.125023

Pharris, A. B., Munoz, R. T., Kratz, J., & Hellman, C. M. (2023). Hope as a buffer to suicide attempts among adolescents with depression. *Journal of School Health, 93*(6), 494–499. https://doi.org/10.1111/josh.13278.

Russinova, Z. (1999). Providers' hope-inspiring competence as a factor optimizing psychiatric rehabilitation. *Journal of Rehabilitation, 65*(4), 50–57.

Snyder, C. R., Hoza, B., Pelham, W. E., et al. (1997). The development and validation of the Children's Hope Scale. *Journal of Pediatric Psychology, 22*(3), 399–421. https://doi.org/10.1093/jpepsy/22.3.399.

Chapter 10

How Solution Focused Practice aligns with the principles of procedural justice and can change frontline policing for the better

Emma Burns

The views expressed in this chapter reflect the author's personal views and do not necessarily indicate either a New Zealand Police or a New Zealand government position.

Many countries rely heavily on their police service to respond to persons in the community who are experiencing significant mental health crises. New Zealand Police, like many of their international counterparts, experience high levels of calls for service to mentally distressed individuals.

In a news release dated August 2024, New Zealand Police Commissioner Andrew Coster noted that

> mental health demand accounted for 11 percent of calls to our Emergency Communications Centre in the year to May 2024. Police receive one mental health-related call every seven minutes, taking up about half a million hours of Police frontline time per year. Of those events, only five percent had a criminal element and 11% of calls are coded P1 and are given a priority response.

With persons experiencing mental distress or crisis relying on a rapid response from police, it is critical that officers are adequately trained and equipped to respond to individuals in a way that reduces risk, protects personal dignity, and connects the person to the right service as quickly as possible. It is also important that police can make decisions in a timely manner and that these are free of bias or prejudice.

There has been long-standing unrest regarding the extent to which police are involved in mental health response. From November 2024, new, higher thresholds for a police response to mental health callouts will be introduced. Calls for service that fall short of this threshold will not be attended by police but directed to more appropriate services.

Additionally, New Zealand's Mental Health Minister Matt Doocey has noted that people seeking crisis support could become further distressed by the presence

DOI: 10.4324/9781003519225-10

of a uniformed officer. 'People in mental distress are not criminals,' he said. 'Those seeking assistance deserve a mental health response, rather than a criminal justice response.'[1]

Furthermore, Health NZ chief executive Margie Apa has noted that proposed changes were about 'getting the balance right' and there were times when a health response was more desirable.[2] For example, 'the potential stigma experienced by a distressed person waiting in an emergency department for a mental health assessment can be exacerbated if they are accompanied by Police.'[3]

Enabling the frontline

While a clear delineation is made between the role of a police officer and the public mental health sector, in practice, this line can become blurred. The New Zealand Mental Health Act gives specific powers to constabulary members, predominantly regarding the apprehension, detention, and transport of persons believed to be mentally disordered (Mental Health (Compulsory Assessment and Treatment) Act 1992). Detention may last for no longer than six hours. As with many other countries, this can result in officers being occupied for many hours, resulting in a decreased capacity to focus on core policing activities. Accordingly, the ability to respond rapidly and appropriately is critical for officers in order to resolve these calls in a safe and ethical manner.

Introducing Solution Focused Practice

The author began working for New Zealand Police in 2010 and was introduced to the Solution Focused approach approximately 12 months later. At that time, she was working with young offenders and their families, with many of these young people also being under mental health services. Rapidly, it became evident that a Solution Focused way of engaging not only led to progress in a timelier manner but also supported a more optimistic, respectful, and collaborative way of working with those in the community.

Since that time, interest has built for utilising this approach more broadly in the organisation, both in training police in public interactions, and the approach to leadership development. Examples will be given later in this chapter, highlighting the difference the Solution Focused approach can make in these public interactions, not only for the person in distress but for the officers themselves – their confidence, morale, and job satisfaction.

The link between Solution Focused Practice and procedural justice

In Plato's vision of a perfect society – in a republic that honors the core of democracy – the greatest amount of power is given to those called the Guardians.

Only those with the most impeccable character are chosen to bear the responsibility of protecting the democracy.

(Nila & Covey, 2008)

The 'Guardian' mindset has humanity and humane interactions at its very core, with a focus on ethical behaviour and ethical decision-making processes. This is consistent with the stance of community policing and the notion that there should ideally be a partnership between a community and its police service. These ideas are consistent with the New Zealand Police Commissioner's vision of 'policing by consent' and the stance of 'doing with' rather than 'doing to' persons and whānau.[4] By way of contrast, the very term 'law enforcement' evokes a sense of significant power imbalance and suggests the use of coercive control.

The most significant determinant of the level of trust and confidence enjoyed by a nation's police service is the public perception of the degree to which police uphold procedural justice.

Procedural justice should be understood as both the evidence of and the hope for processes that resolve disputes and allocate resources fairly. It speaks to four key principles, often referred to as the four 'pillars' of procedural justice. These are:

- Voice – people have the opportunity to tell their story, to be listened to, and to have confidence that those in authority will genuinely consider this before making any decisions.
- Neutrality (often referred to as impartiality) – authority figures are seen as impartial and principled decision-makers, with transparency of process and free from bias.
- Respect – people feel as though they are treated with respect by agency representatives, and they believe that their dignity and rights are upheld throughout the processes.
- Trust – authorities are seen as trustworthy, sincere, authentic, and striving to do what is right for everyone.

It follows logically that a police service that is seen to demonstrate these principles of procedural justice will enjoy stronger relationships with their communities, earn the trust and confidence of the public, and be supported and assisted by the public to protect the communities they serve.

Fundamental to procedural justice is the degree to which a police service enables and supports staff to respond to and resolve incidents in a way that upholds the principles outlined previously.

Police are called to respond to a wide range of situations in the community, ranging from incidents that are relatively simple and quickly resolved to more serious and complex events that may include significant threats to life and the potential to turn deadly. Mental health crises may be resolved in a timely manner, or they may escalate to a more serious encounter. The Solution Focused approach has been found to contribute significantly to de-escalation, a critical component in the resolution of incidents.

Changing mindsets

New Zealand Police is a large organisation, employing close to 16,000 staff. Of these, approximately 11,000 are constabulary (sworn) staff. New Zealand Police also employs approximately 5,000 civilian (non-sworn) staff across the organisation. Accordingly, any project designed to shift mindset or practice represents a significant change programme. In a fast-paced and rapidly evolving environment, this can be challenging.

One of the tenets of Solution Focused Practice is that small steps can lead to big changes (De Shazer et al., 2007). Over time, police became curious about the progress being made by the young people and families I had been working with, which led to a shift in my work towards providing training and mentoring for staff interested in using the approach. An evaluation took place in 2020, which demonstrated that officers who had received two 90-minute training sessions reported better engagement and higher job satisfaction.

In recent years, the approach has been slowly integrated into other parts of the organisation. Particularly relevant to this chapter is the training of police recruits in using the Solution Focused approach with suicidal persons. In this training, recruits learn how to use Haesun Moon's Dialogic Orientation Quadrant to be more intentional regarding their focus and questioning (Moon, 2020).

In addition to the improved public interactions, police report an increased sense of having made a difference for people and that this style of engagement created the opportunity to get to know 'the whole person,' not merely the person in the context of the incident they were involved in. Solution Focused questions regarding what *better* looks like led to discussion about coping and resources, who their support people are, and help rapidly to build relationships. The distressed person in crisis is seen as a fellow human, not a job to be resolved. This provides a strong counter against the organisational risks of dehumanisation, for example, falling into the habit of referring to a mentally distressed person as a '1M' (the police code for mental health calls). It also leads to more balanced information being entered into the national intelligence system and careful thinking applied to the use of mental health flags.

Ethical practice

As mentioned in an earlier section, upholding procedural justice is vital in policing. New officers are now being trained in this, including in a framework underpinned by Solution Focused principles aligned with the four pillars of procedural justice.

It is recognised that one of the greatest ethical risks for police is moral disengagement. This is defined as the process where an individual or group of people distance themselves from the normal or accepted ethical standards of behaviour and believe that certain unethical behaviours are justified. Moral disengagement is a process that is understood to take place via several mechanisms. In the policing context, one of the key mechanisms by which moral disengagement occurs is dehumanisation – that is, the process by which a person or group of people is denied 'humanness' or human attributes. The person is no longer viewed as a worthy human with hopes, feelings, and value but objectified as a lesser being with negligible inherent worth. This view then justifies treating that person or group of people with less empathy, compassion, or respect, and in the extreme, leads to justification of abuse or violence.

A potential defence against unethical decision-making is the selection of a style of engagement that militates against dehumanisation. Many of the person-centred approaches that encourage a focus on the person rather than the problem offer some degree of protection against dehumanisation. However, police officers are not therapists, and many of these approaches are time-consuming and require multiple sessions in order to make progress.

The Solution Focused approach is a simple approach to engagement that offers many benefits to the police setting. Not only does it uphold police values and the mana[5] of individuals and whānau, its focus on a person's aspirations and strengths is inherently incompatible with dehumanisation – quite simply, it is not possible to speak with someone about their values, abilities, and hopes and simultaneously view them as devoid of human attributes or worth. Additionally, this style of engagement is consistent with the principles of procedural justice, thereby creating a very different dynamic and increasing trust and confidence. Indeed, procedural justice is amplified by a Solution Focused approach because offenders are more likely to comply with decisions if they believe the decision was made in a fair manner. This enhances the credibility of the justice system as a whole and upholds therapeutic jurisprudence – the principle that if people in the justice system are treated with fairness and dignity, this will have a positive impact on their wellbeing.

Additionally, it is the author's experience and belief that engaging with communities utilising a Solution Focused approach increases the likelihood that policing will embody fairness, inclusivity, and decision-making that is impartial and free of prejudice or bias. The Solution Focused approach to interactions invites an understanding of the whole person – not merely their identity as 'mental health client,' 'victim,' or 'offender.'

Changing practice

The following case examples represent excellent application of the Solution Focused approach in responding to calls for service involving members of the public with a significant history of mental ill-health and suicide attempts.

This first example is from a young police recruit who had learned how to use the approach with suicidal persons during a 90-minute session titled 'Conversations that Create Hope.' The incident described took place during deployment week – this falls in Week 17 of the 20-week residential learning programme. She was called to respond to a middle-aged father of five children who had earlier that day been stopped by his family from jumping off a high building. Later that evening, he had left his address, and police were searching for him.

There was a suicide job. The mother called [to tell us] . . . that he's going to commit suicide. They had already stopped him jumping out a high window that day. They have train tracks running behind their property. It was, like, nine o'clock at night. And we're like, okay, we've got to check the train tracks.

I was with two other officers . . . . We had to jump over a fence and, you know, it was just like crazy . . . we had to run along the track lines, get a hold of KiwiRail to tell them to stop the trains. And I spotted a little light of someone . . . . He was lying on the train track, and I was like, he's over there, and then I just had to run to him, and we just had to talk him off. And about maybe a minute later, the train came past. So, it was a crazy moment, but . . . I was like, wow. Like . . . it just [motivated] me even more.

I felt prepared for that moment personally because I was in that mindset. Like, okay, someone's life is at risk. Just got to do whatever we can.

At college, we had a lesson on how to talk to someone who's feeling suicidal, [having] suicidal thoughts. That kicked in, and how I talked to them and approached them, what things to say, what things not to say. And, yeah, all that training definitely kicked in.

That session, I will say, is really good to see how we would approach someone who has suicidal thoughts or who's going to jump off a bridge. What led you to this? But then, looking for his reasons to live, and he said, 'Well, I have five kids.' And I was like, 'You have five kids?' And we just talked about them. It was relatable to him. I think we connected on that. But that whole session at college just kicked in, and I was like, wow.

Like, you are going come up to these situations where obviously you're talking to someone who's about to end their life, and how would you approach that? How would you speak to them? Or what would you say to them? And you don't want to say the wrong thing, but this session helped me know what to focus on – how to listen for his reasons for living and to engage with him in a way that reduced his agitation and distress so that we could get him to safety.

We were taught how to do that in the session. All these pieces coming together and actually seeing it practically and doing it practically just instilled even more confidence in me.

I feel like that was an important moment, like a pinpoint moment for me in my deployment. In my whole career and obviously in life because that is someone's life that I possibly saved with only a few minutes to spare [before the train came].

It also highlighted the risk . . . to us as police officers: where we put ourselves at risk to save another . . . . And the sergeant highlighted that when we got back to the station because, obviously, we had contacted KiwiRail to stop the trains, but there must have been a miscommunication because they didn't stop it in time. And if that came maybe 20 seconds earlier, possibly that guy's life ended, [but it] put the officers at risk as well. That session maybe saved more than one life.

The second example is from a Senior Sergeant working as the Area Manager for Police Custody Units. He has over 28 years of experience in frontline policing, including roles as a public safety officer, operational dog handler, search and rescue team member, and response manager.

In 2019, I moved from being an operational dog handler to that of a section supervisor. During my time as a dog handler, I had encountered many people suffering from a range of mental conditions, but it wasn't until I became a supervisor that I began to get up close and personal with many of these people.

I recall an incident where a young male had an argument with his partner and during this had picked up a knife and threatened to kill himself in front of her. Naturally, police were called, and I was first on the scene. The conversation, quite rightly, centred around the incident but didn't offer any form of solution or help, even though police had a Prevention First approach to anything and everything. Our conversation was rather invasive and centred around his actions of the day, and I could see we were getting nowhere, and he was getting worked up.

Soon after this, I contacted Emma, and she spoke to me about Solution Focused [Practice] and then provided training to myself and my team. This meant that police had to change their mindset and focus more on 'what keeps people here' rather than on what is making them do what they do. The logic and reasoning were obvious but foreign to us as I had never been exposed to this.

Sometime later, I had the opportunity to put this into practise when a young lady by the name of Samantha (not her real name) had attempted to harm herself by walking into the surf at a nearby beach. Samantha had an extensive history of mental health concerns, including borderline personality disorder and frequent suicide attempts.

I spoke with Samantha at her home address, meaning I had limited police powers to deal with this in the usual manner. This was a blessing in disguise as it meant I could sit down with her and simply talk. Initially, Samantha didn't want to listen and stormed in and out of the room, but each time I focused on something positive, and I guess she saw that this wasn't the typical police visit. Perhaps this officer did really care, and she was right.

Samantha sat down, and we began to talk. She led the conversation and told me about the events of the day and what had happened at the beach. She also disclosed that she had tried to self-harm several times, and that was my 'in.' My first reply to her was, 'Samantha – you are still here, so there is something that is keeping you here. What might that be?'

She disclosed that during her latest relationship, she had grown fondly of the young child and became like a mother figure, and the young child was only being raised by their father. She went on to say that she loved the child so much that she couldn't bear thinking of the child being left alone without her around anymore, and that was what was keeping her here. The issue, though, was that she wasn't really dealing with the relationship break-up that well. As the conversation progressed, it moved into where she may receive the help she needs so she can navigate this safely and come out the other side, knowing that the relationship is over but that she could still see the young child and continue to be a positive role model.

I left the address feeling rather happy with myself and that I had achieved something without having to expose her to the normal mental health procedures that police follow. This was more personal, and it involved the three of us – Samantha, her grandmother, and me.

Later that day, while on my way home, Samantha rang me and thanked me for the time I had spent with her. I can still recall the time and place and even point out where I pulled over to speak with her. That is how memorable the phone call was. Something like that had never happened to me before.

I have since moved on but have taken the skills I learnt through Emma and the Solution Focused approach into other areas of my work. I am now working in a Police custody unit, and what better place to again use these skills, especially with our youth. Who knows, maybe the conversations I have with them may in some way stop them from coming back into my world.

A third and final example comes from an officer tasked with executing one of the most challenging and, at times, emotive jobs police are called to attend – the uplift of a child from the family. In this case, the father from whom the child was to be removed was well known to police – he had an extensive offending history and was president of one of the chapters of a prominent gang in New Zealand. Additionally, he was a New Zealand Māori male, and it is well documented that indigenous cultures are often overrepresented in 'use of force' statistics. The author was privileged to be able to reunite these two men several years later and was curious about what made this interaction so powerful. The following is a summary of what took place that night.

The attending officers knew this man's history and the level of potential risk involved; thus, part of attending the job was completing a risk assessment. However, one of the officers consciously decided to avoid a confrontational approach, which would likely have set the foundation for an escalation. Instead, he approached this as humanely as possible, understanding that the man was about to have his child removed from his care and that it would be distressing for all. The focus, therefore, became less about getting the job done and more about carrying it out with empathy and humanity. What made a difference was the follow-up contact. After the child had been removed, the officer returned to check in on the man, letting him know that his son was safe and on the way to his mother, explaining what had happened and what his rights were. Essentially, this interaction changed from being between a police officer and an offender to one between fellow humans. What the officer did not realise until approximately seven years later, when they were reunited, was that this second interaction had prevented a suicide, and created the first stepping stone for a complete life transformation from a violent, drug-selling gang president to a man who serves the community, has adopted children and become the pastor of a church.

Concluding remarks

Policing is a demanding career – both physically and emotionally – and it carries very real risks to physical and psychological safety. The threats to wellness are well documented, with more recent literature highlighting the moral risks of policing and the link between high levels of trauma, moral disengagement, and unethical practice (Blumberg et al., 2020). However, these real and ever-present dangers are largely unknown to the public, who only see the disturbing outcomes when things go wrong. These adverse incidents are often accompanied by extensive coverage, both via official news reporting and on social media. Incidents like these often result in public anger, erosion of trust and confidence, or calls such as 'defund the police.' The countless examples of ethical and helpful interactions between police and members of the public rarely see the light of day, as they are not deemed newsworthy.

Additionally, the author often remarks when delivering training to police recruits that nobody calls 111 to report having a good day. Police assistance is required by people who often present at their worst, on their worst days. Adopting a Solution Focused stance enables officers to understand that the people they are called to assist are agitated, dysregulated, and unable to manage their situation. Asking Solution Focused questions not only assists with de-escalation and risk reduction but also creates an entirely different dialogue. This was summed up perfectly by a very new constable who, having received one 90-minute training session, attended a family harm incident and asked the following question – 'We come to your house a lot – what would we see if we came on a good day?' The respect and genuine curiosity conveyed in such a simple question changed the entire trajectory of that incident, as well as the relationship between police and that family.

The Solution Focused approach has been shown to be protective against burnout in child protection workers (Medina & Beyebach, 2014). This is a group that shares similar risk factors to police. It is the author's experience and observation that when police services are trained in Solution Focused Practice this can lead to better engagement, greater procedural justice, and stronger police-citizen relationships, and these things themselves lead to better outcomes for our communities, as well as greater public trust and confidence.

Notes

1 New approach to mental health calls welcomed | Beehive.govt.nz.
2 https://www.rnz.co.nz/news/national/526608/police-unveil-plan-to-reduce-attendance-at-mental-health-call-outs.

3   https://www.1news.co.nz/2024/08/30/changes-coming-to-how-police-respond-to-mental-health-callouts/.
4   Whānau is often translated as 'family,' but its meaning is more complex. It includes physical, emotional, and spiritual dimensions and is based on whakapapa. Whānau can be multi-layered, flexible, and dynamic. Whānau is based on a Māori and a tribal world-view. It is through the whānau that values, histories, and traditions from the ancestors are adapted for the contemporary world.
5   Mana is a Māori word that refers to a person's prestige, power, status, and influence.

References

Blumberg, D., Papazoglou, K., & Schlosser, M. (2020). Organizational solutions to the moral risks of policing. *International Journal of Environmental Research and Public Health, 17*. https://doi.org/10.3390/ijerph17207461.

De Shazer, S., Dolan, Y., Korman, H., Trepper, T., McCollum, E., & Berg, I. (2007). *More than Miracles: The state of the art of solution-focussed brief therapy*. Routledge.

den Heyer, G. (2021), Risk and protective factors for post-traumatic stress among New Zealand police personnel: A cross sectional study. *Policing: An International Journal, 44*(5), 909–925. https://doi.org/10.1108/PIJPSM-01-2021-0001.

Medina, A., & Beyebach, M. (2014). The impact of solution-focused training on professionals' beliefs, practices and burnout of child protection workers in Tenerife Island. *Child Care in Practice, 20*(1), 7–36. https://doi.org/10.1080/13575279.2013.847058.

Moon, H. (2020). Coaching: Using ordinary words in extraordinary ways. In S. McNamee, M. Gergen, C. Camargo-Borges, & E. Rasera (Eds.), *The sage handbook of social constructionist practice* (pp. 246–257). Sage. https://doi.org/10.4135/9781529714326.

Nila, M., & Covey, S. (2008). *The nobility of policing*. Franklin Quest.

Chapter 11

Solution Focused Practice can help us to deliver a more inclusive and empowering psychiatry

Nektarios Kouvarakis

National Health Service (NHS) difficulties are frequently highlighted in the UK media, especially so in the wake of the Covid-19 pandemic and annual winter crises. NHS mental health services have their difficulties, too, competing as they are for dwindling resources. When I arrived from Greece in 2003 to continue my training in psychiatry, I was in awe of how advanced mental health services were at the time, offering a variety of special interventions and expertise. There were no significant staffing issues; inpatient beds were readily available, and I felt optimistic services could only improve. However, over the following 20 years, I witnessed reforms which have led to the current mental health landscape: a radical reduction of inpatient bed availability; patients waiting in A&E for days and occasionally weeks before admission; acute staffing crises, with staff being overworked and overstressed; and patients feeling more 'managed' than 'treated'.

We must relieve the pressure on mental health services amid an ever-growing NHS fiscal demand and also try to deliver the government's aim to achieve parity of esteem between physical and mental health services (Department of Health, 2011). Clinicians and policymakers generally agree on the importance of mental wellbeing to overall health and the need for equitable resource allocation. However, staffing and financial issues continue to prevent improvement.

In this context, the difficulties in providing quality mental health interventions in a timely way are obvious. Trained workers are not always available; several months- (if not years-) long waiting lists prevent patients from accessing treatment and day-to-day clinical contact is reduced from an opportunity for a meaningful therapeutic step to a fire-fighting exercise. This increases the likelihood of inefficient interventions and patients not progressing, as well as 'revolving door' admissions which manage to solve one crisis just before the next one arises.

This is where the value of the Solution Focused (SF) approach becomes apparent. Several qualities, characteristics and principles of the Solution Focused philosophy are well suited to facilitate improvement in healthcare service provision and will be highlighted in this chapter. I have sought to concentrate on a small number of issues which serve as examples to highlight how Solution Focused Practice (SFP) can be very useful in addressing ongoing challenges.

DOI: 10.4324/9781003519225-11

Reducing discrimination

Discrimination in the context of mental health crisis has been highlighted in a number of studies and documents, and racialised minorities in the UK are much more likely to be subjected to detention under the Mental Health Act (Gajwani et al., 2016). This said, protecting human rights and reducing discrimination is central to contemporary mental health policies. The Equality Act 2010 consolidates anti-discrimination laws, ensuring that individuals with mental health conditions are protected from unfair treatment. Campaigns like *Time to Change* have played a significant role in challenging stigma and promoting understanding, contributing to cultural shifts in how mental ill-health is perceived (Time to Change, 2020). Furthermore, the UK's ratification of the United Nations Convention on the Rights of Persons with Disabilities underscores a commitment to upholding the rights of those with mental health conditions (United Nations, 2006).

The use of SFP during clinical encounters appears to have advantages in reducing discrimination. Specifically, Solution Focused philosophy places the client at the helm of managing their difficulties and finding solutions; it does not seek to impose any agenda on the client and generally leads from 'one step behind' (Cantwell & Holmes, 1994). This allows the client to express their own ideas and goals (Ratner et al., 2012) and serves to empower disadvantaged clients to express their hopes and wishes without systems-driven pressures imposing a pre-packaged set of outcomes – outcomes which often do not take personal and cultural needs into account.

Case Study 1

Thabo (pseudonym) is a 30-year-old African man diagnosed with bipolar disorder. He believes in communicating with his ancestors – a common practice in his culture known as ancestral veneration. This belief system includes rituals and dreams through which he feels guided and supported by his ancestors. He is currently an inpatient, has improved in his mood and seeks therapy to manage mood swings but is hesitant because previous healthcare providers dismissed his cultural beliefs as delusions, worsening his mistrust and feelings of discrimination. He has the following discussion with me:

Nektarios (N):   Thabo, I'm glad you decided to spend some time with me discussing your progress. What are your best hopes for our meeting today?

Thabo (T):   I want to find ways to manage my mood swings so I can take better care of my family. I also hope to speak freely without being judged for my beliefs. (*Thabo is highlighting his goals and leading the interview*)

N: What would it look like if you were managing your moods in a way that feels right to you?

T:	I would feel more balanced. I could recognise when a mood shift is coming and maybe do something to prevent it from taking over.
N:	Can you tell me about a time when you were able to sense a mood shift coming and managed it effectively? (*Focusing on T's resources and strengths*)
T:	Yes, last month I felt myself getting anxious. I performed a calming ritual my grandmother taught me, and it helped me stay grounded.
N:	That's wonderful. It sounds like your grandmother's teachings are a valuable resource for you. How else have your ancestral practices helped you? (*Avoiding medicalisation*)
T:	They give me strength and guidance. When I honour my ancestors, I feel supported and less alone.
N:	I appreciate you sharing that with me. Your connection with your ancestors is an important part of your life. How can we incorporate this connection into strategies for managing your moods?
T:	Maybe we can create a plan that includes my rituals and respects my beliefs.
N:	Absolutely. Let's work together to build a plan that combines your cultural practices with techniques to help you maintain balance. What steps would you like to take first? (*Working collaboratively*)
T:	I think setting aside time each day for my rituals would help. Also, learning more about how to recognise early signs of mood changes.
N:	On a scale of zero to ten, where zero means you have no control over your mood swings and ten means you feel fully in control, where would you say you are now?
T:	Maybe a four.
N:	What makes it a four and not a lower number?
T:	Because I already have some tools, like my rituals, that help me sometimes.
N:	How would you know if it was a five or a six? (*Use of scaling questions*)
T:	I could try to be more consistent with my rituals and perhaps learn other techniques to stay calm.

The questions that are asked support Thabo to lead the conversation and draw upon his cultural strengths. As his psychiatrist, I am able to demonstrate respect for his beliefs by integrating them into the therapeutic process rather than dismissing them as symptoms of his illness. Patient-led solution finding is essential to the Solution Focused approach.

Outcomes

- Improved trust: Thabo feels heard and respected, increasing his trust in the therapeutic relationship
- Cultural integration: incorporating his ancestral practices enhances his engagement and provides culturally relevant coping mechanisms
- Reduced discrimination: acknowledging his beliefs as cultural rather than pathological reduces feelings of discrimination and stigma
- Enhanced self-efficacy: focusing on his strengths and past successes boosts his confidence in managing his mood swings

Legal, ethical and human rights considerations

The new Mental Health Bill, introduced in late 2024 and derived from the Wessely Review (Independent Review of the Mental Health Act 1983, 2018), demonstrates further legislative efforts to prioritise more independence, autonomy and anti-discrimination for people experiencing mental ill-health.

The Wessely Review promotes the following principles:

1 Choice and autonomy – ensuring service users' views and choices are respected
2 Least restriction – ensuring the Act's powers are used in the least restrictive way
3 Therapeutic benefit – ensuring patients are supported to get better so they can be discharged from the Act
4 The person as an individual – ensuring patients are viewed and treated as rounded individuals

From my clinical point of view, the utilisation of SFP is inherently advantageous in achieving more choice and autonomy as well as treating the person as an individual. It emphasises the use of the person's strengths and encourages them to find their own solutions creatively. This can reduce the need for enforcing, restrictive practices. In his chapter highlighting his application of SFP to the role of the Approved Mental Health Professional, Nick Perry will look at this in more detail and the way in which SFP can support anti-racist practice.

Personalised care

It makes sense that adapting plans to personal needs (we could call them 'best hopes') can improve overall outcomes for patients. This requirement was identified in the Five Year Forward View for Mental Health, which outlined a comprehensive approach to improving services, focusing on early intervention, integrated care and person-centred practices (NHS England, 2016).

Legislative changes, such as the amendments to the Mental Health Act in 2007 (with more due very soon), have modernised the legal framework and enhanced patient rights and safeguards. The introduction of the Care Act 2014 further solidified the rights of individuals to receive personalised care that promotes independence and well-being. SFP is well placed to deliver on such aims. It holds that people are the experts on their own lives and difficulties and that they possess the inner resources and strengths necessary to solve their own problems. Healthcare professionals act merely as facilitators, helping people to tap into these abilities. Extrapolating from Evan George's chapter in this book, if services follow this way of thinking, they will begin to conform to client needs, not the other way round.

Case Study 2

Alex (pseudonym) is a 22-year-old man who suffers with schizophrenia, currently in remission. He attends an appointment with his psychiatrist for a review of his progress, in which he appears anxious. He has previously discussed with his psychiatrist that he is not good with words and does not want to have counselling or psychotherapy for his anxiety at this stage, but he recognises the need to be able to express himself:

Clinician (C):	Hi Alex, it's good to see you today. What are your best hopes from our conversation?
Alex (A):	I guess I want to feel less anxious and find ways to express myself better, as we discussed before; I still do not want to have talking therapy sessions.
C:	Imagine that tonight you go to sleep, and a miracle happens overnight – the kind of miracle that makes your life feel just right. When you wake up tomorrow, what would be the first signs that tell you things have improved? (Use of miracle question)
A:	I would wake up feeling calm, not worried about things. I'd feel motivated to do something I enjoy, like painting.
C:	Oh, I did not know you enjoyed painting! (Identifying past successes and exceptions)
A:	I used to be good at it at school. I did not enjoy other classes and art was my favourite subject. I was stressed with maths and English, but painting was very calming for me.
C:	What was it about those art classes that made you feel at ease? (Emphasis on strengths)
A:	I think it was the freedom to express myself and the support from my art teacher, who understood me.
C:	Well, there is a local art group led by an artist who is also a therapist! Would you be interested in exploring that as a way to express yourself without having to talk about your difficulties?
A:	Maybe it is a good idea; you know I don't enjoy deep conversations about me and my problems.
C:	On a scale of zero to ten, where zero means you're feeling extremely anxious and ten means you're feeling completely at ease,

where would you say you are today? (*Scaling questions*)

A: Maybe a six.

C: What makes it a six and not lower, say, a four?

A: Well, I'm thinking about the possibility of joining these art sessions. I remember it was nice painting with others when I was on the ward a couple of years ago.

C: That's great to hear. If you found yourself at seven, how would you know? What would tell you?

A: Actually attending the art group and seeing if it helps me feel more relaxed. I will not know until I do it.

C: What do you expect might happen at the art session that could make that difference for you?

A: Being able to paint again with guidance from someone experienced and maybe connecting with others who share similar interests.

C: It sounds like painting is a significant positive outlet for you. How would you feel about incorporating these art sessions into your care plan?

A: I would really like that. Maybe it could help me manage my anxiety.

C: What steps can we take to make this happen?

A: I could sign up for the next session and make it a regular part of my routine.

C: What might get in the way of you attending these sessions, and how can we plan to overcome those obstacles?

A: Sometimes, my anxiety makes it hard to go out. Maybe we could arrange for someone to go with me the first few times.

C: That's a good idea. Is there someone you trust who could accompany you?

A: My sister is very supportive; I'm sure she would help.

C: It's wonderful that you're taking proactive steps and that you have support from your sister. Attending these art sessions could be a significant step toward feeling more at ease. How confident do you feel about following through with this plan?

A: I'm feeling pretty hopeful – maybe seven out of ten.

C: That's encouraging. How could we improve on that?

A: Maybe, if I could meet the artist beforehand, so I know what to expect.

C: I can help arrange an introductory meeting if you'd like.

A: Yes, that would help a lot.

Outcomes:

- Promoting autonomy and collaboration: the discussion is led by Alex. He is finding solutions to his own difficulties, looking in his past life and taking the expert role on how to move things forward
- Alex's care is adapted to him: he identifies old strengths, and solutions are adapted to his needs
- Improved engagement: Alex's engagement is improved by his agency. He feels validated in expressing his ideas and using his own strengths. As a result, he is more likely to participate in developing his care plans and achieve an improved prognosis

Reducing stigma

Stigma remains a significant barrier to seeking help and recovering from mental health conditions. National campaigns, educational programs and policy initiatives aim to change public perceptions, promote understanding and encourage openness about mental health. By normalising mental health discussions, we can begin to dismantle prejudices and support individuals in accessing the care they need (Slade, 2009; Department of Health, 2011). SFP is non-pathologising and avoids focusing on the medical model, which, in my clinical opinion, can enhance stigma. In SFP, the focus is on helping the client find a solution to their problem, not analyse their pre-existing conditions. Solutions could be medical or not. By not fixating on solutions that are rigidly connected to established psychiatric diagnoses, we can help clients to feel listened to and less stigmatised. SFP sees individuals as capable of change regardless of their challenges or the mental health crises they might be grappling with.

Case Study 3

Jacob (pseudonym), a 32-year-old man diagnosed with schizophrenia, has recently entered a period of relative stability following a challenging psychotic episode. Despite fewer acute symptoms, Jacob experiences persistent anxiety, low self-esteem and internalised stigma related to his diagnosis. He worries about how others view him, leading to isolation and reluctance to engage in community activities. The purpose of SFP is not to dwell excessively on problems but to collaborate with the patient to identify existing strengths and resources and envision a hopeful future (Franklin et al., 2016; de Shazer & Dolan, 2007).

C: Jacob, I'm glad you're here today. What are your best hopes from our conversation? (*Engagement and best hopes*)

J: I'd like to feel less afraid about what people think of me. I want to feel more at ease, maybe join the gym again – like I used to before I got really unwell. (*Jacob articulates his own goals, being an expert in his own life; feels empowered and counters stigma*; Franklin et al., 2012)

> *C:* If a miracle happened overnight and you woke up feeling more confident, what would be the first thing you'd notice? (*Preferred future: the clinician guides Jacob to envisage a scenario in which stigma and fear are less dominant; the focus is on the future that Jacob wants, not past problems;* Gingerich & Peterson, 2013)
>
> *J:* I'd wake up looking forward to the day. Maybe I'd feel excited about going for a run. I'd feel like my diagnosis didn't define me and that other people just saw me as Jacob, the guy who loves sports.
>
> *C:* Can you remember a time, however short, when you felt more accepted and less anxious about how others saw you? (*Identifying resources and exceptions*)
>
> *J:* Five years ago, I was in a five-a-side football team. They just treated me like anyone else, passing the ball, chatting about technique after the game; I was one of the lads. (*Normalised and valued activities which reduce internalised stigma*)

With this, a plan emerges: Jacob will explore sports activities and exercise groups in the community, starting from a walking group and moving to table tennis and football. By building on his interests and previous positive experiences, SFP promotes environments where Jacob sees himself as more than a diagnosis. This counters stigma by highlighting personal competence and social connection.

Cost-effective care

As Guy Shennan's chapter encourages us, SFP can be used in single, one-off clinical encounters. Every session with a client, be it in A&E, in a crisis assessment in the community or during Mental Health Act work, can be an opportunity for meaningful interventions, creating a basis for solutions to be found by the client. Both clients and healthcare staff can have confidence that one-off encounters can have a meaningful therapeutic effect; this is immensely rewarding to staff, and clients can start to feel appreciated and empowered rather than the opposite.

Case Study 4

Emma (pseudonym) is a 28-year-old woman who arrives at the Accident & Emergency (A&E) Department expressing feelings of moderate depression, but she has no plans or intent to harm herself. She is overwhelmed by her symptoms but is hesitant about hospital admission. The clinician aims to use SF questions during this single contact to help Emma develop a care plan that allows her to manage her depression in the community, thus avoiding hospitalisation:

> *Clinician (C):* Hi Emma, . . . What are your best hopes from our conversation today?
>
> *Emma (E):* I just want to feel a bit better and find a way to cope with everything that's going on . . .

C: If we were to have a helpful conversation today, and you left feeling more hopeful, what would be different for you?

E: I might have a clearer idea of how to handle my feelings and maybe some steps I can take to start feeling like myself again. (*Patient is setting goals*)

C: Can you tell me about a time in the past when you felt better or were able to cope with difficult feelings?

E: A few months ago, I was feeling down, but I started going for walks with a friend, and it really helped. (*Identifying patient resources*)

C: That's great to hear. What was it about those walks that made a difference for you?

E: Being active and having someone to talk to made me feel less alone.

C: On a scale of zero to ten, where zero means things are as bad as they could be and ten means you've recovered and feel back to your usual self, where do you see yourself now?

E: Maybe a three.

C: What makes it a three and not lower?

E: I still have some support from my family, and I can get out of bed most days . . .

C: If you found yourself just one point up the scale, how would you know? What might you notice yourself doing?

E: I think I would be reconnecting with my friend and starting those walks again could help.

C: That sounds like a positive step. What else might contribute to moving up the scale?

E: Perhaps talking to a counsellor or joining a support group. (*Patient finding suitable solutions*)

C: It seems like you have some ideas about what could help you feel better. How do you feel about creating a plan together to incorporate these activities? (*Collaborative approach*)

E: I would like that. Having a plan might make things feel more manageable.

C: You've mentioned some effective strategies you've used before, like walking with a friend and seeking support. It's clear you have strengths and resources to draw upon. How confident do you feel about taking these steps?

E: I'm a bit nervous, but I think I can do it with some support.

C: Let's outline the steps you can take. You can contact your friend to schedule regular walks. Reach out to a counsellor – I can provide you with contact information for community mental health

	services. Inform your family about your plan so they can support you. Give you a point of contact in case you need additional help. How does this plan sound to you?
E:	It sounds helpful. I feel better having a plan.

By using SF questions, the clinician helps Emma to:

- Recognise her existing strengths and resources, such as her supportive family and previous positive experiences
- Visualise a preferred future, motivating her to take actionable steps
- Develop a practical care plan that leverages community resources and personal relationships
- Feel empowered and hopeful, reducing the immediate risk and avoiding hospital admission

Conclusion

I hope the clinical examples in this chapter highlight the strengths of Solution Focused Practice and give insight into the rationale for it becoming more prominent in modern mental health service provision – particularly for people in mental health crisis. My personal experience of using the approach has convinced me of its value in the recovery-oriented forensic mental health service where I practice.

Going forward, further work on the economic evaluation of its effectiveness, inclusion of SFP in training curricula and continuing professional development programs and further development of the evidence base in a variety of settings can develop its usefulness in helping patients achieve better outcomes. Common sense dictates that a treatment philosophy which is encouraging patients to find solutions based on their own personal strengths rather than dwelling on past difficulties and deficits is inherently advantageous at a time when the UK government is legislating for practitioners to provide less restrictive, less discriminatory and more personalised care.

References

Cantwell, P., & Holmes, S. (1994). Social construction: A paradigm shift for systemic therapy and training. *Australian and New Zealand Journal of Family Therapy, 15*, 17–26. https://doi.org/10.1002/j.1467–8438.1994.tb00978.x.

Care Act. (2014). *Care Act 2014*.

de Shazer, S., & Dolan, Y. (2007). *More than Miracles: The state of the art of solution-focused brief therapy*. Haworth Press.

Franklin, C., Trepper, T. S., Gingerich, W., & McCollum, E. (2012). *Solution-focused brief therapy: A handbook of evidence-based practice*. Oxford University Press.

Franklin, C., Zhang, A., Froerer, A., & Johnson, S. (2016). Solution focused brief therapy: A systematic review and meta-summary of process research. *Journal of Marital and Family Therapy, 42*(1), 16–30. https://doi.org/10.1111/jmft.12193.

Gajwani, R., Parsons, H., Birchwood, M., & Singh, S. (2016). Ethnicity and detention: are Black and minority ethnic (BME) groups disproportionately detained under the

Mental Health Act 2007? *Soc Psychiatry Psychiatr Epidemiol, 51*, 703–711. https://doi. org/10.1007/s00127-016-1181-z. Epub 2016 Feb 17.

Gingerich, W. J., & Peterson, L. T. (2013). Effectiveness of solution-focused brief therapy: A systematic qualitative review of controlled outcome studies. *Research on Social Work Practice, 23*(3), 266–283. https://doi.org/10.1177/104973151247085.

Independent Review of the Mental Health Act 1983. (2018). *Modernising the mental health act: Increasing choice, reducing compulsion.* Final Report of the Independent Review of the Mental Health Act 1983.

Mental Health Act. (1983, as amended 2007). *Mental Health Act 2007.*

NHS England. (2016). *The five year forward view for mental health.* NHS England.

Ratner, H., George, E., & Iveson, C. (2012). *Solution focused brief therapy: 100 key points and techniques.* Routledge.

Slade, M. (2009). The contribution of mental health services to recovery. *Journal of Mental Health, 18*(5), 367–371. https://doi.org/10.3109/09638230903191256.

Time to Change. (2020). *Annual report 2019/20. Time to change campaign to end mental health discrimination.* turtl-story-impact-report-20192020.pdf.

United Nations. (2006). *Convention on the rights of persons with disabilities.* United Nations.

Chapter 12

Using Solution Focused Practice to assess and manage suicide risk

Michele Orr

Solution Focused Practice (SFP) is inherently respectful. It acknowledges clients as experts in their own lives: competent and capable of making the changes they want (Ratner et al., 2012). SFP is language-focused, 'hope-inducing' (Fiske, 2008) and communicates compassion and empathy. Suicide prevention researchers (Shand et al., 2018) are clear that clients experiencing suicidal crises need 'empathic and effective care' when in places such as emergency departments (ED). SFP offers just that. Even in times of crisis, the practitioner's role is to tap into hope (Fiske, 2008). When given the privilege to talk with someone who has experienced thoughts of suicide or who has survived a suicide attempt, we need to make good use of it. It may be the one opportunity to make a difference.

SFP is respectful not only inter-personally but also inter-culturally, offering an opportunity to work successfully with minoritized and racialized groups. In SFP, the co-construction of the client's desired outcome is enhanced by the amplification of the cultural resources inherent in their socio-cultural milieu (Lee, 2003).

Research tells us that clients experience positive outcomes when the person seeing them holds hope for them (Blundo et al., 2014). Compared to problem-solving models, SFP is 'laser-focused on hope' (Connie & Froerer, 2023). Even a client's willingness to have a conversation with a helping professional should be acknowledged as a sign of hope.

SFP honours the client's autonomy and agency as they begin to describe their own competence. Answering Solution Focused questions broadens clients' thinking to possibilities other than suicide. They experience a version of themselves with capability and the possibilities of a life worth living.

Trusting SFP in suicidal crisis 'assessment' and within public mental health environments allows the practitioner to develop a realistic understanding of the client and their hopes. SFP can be balanced with a medical model enhancing client safety and wellbeing (Wright et al., 2015). SFP empowers clients and practitioners to make safer decisions (Wright et al., 2015). Although Solution Focused questions are not risk assessment questions, they derive important and sufficient information to complete any mandated risk assessment.

SFP hope-filled conversations (Connie & Froerer, 2023) start by asking, 'What are your best hopes from our conversation today?'. If a client is subject to statutory

DOI: 10.4324/9781003519225-12

requirements and a legal framework, we ask about a client's best hopes within those parameters (Ratner et al., 2012, p. 25). Understanding best hopes and subsequent desired outcomes can help to navigate complex systems: away from areas such as ED or Crisis Team caseloads and towards preferred futures (aka 'discharge pathways').

Clients sometimes answer, 'I don't know', to the questions we ask. We remain quiet, we slow down and wait: giving them more thinking time. Clients considering suicide as an option can experience cognitive constriction. Although there are often time constraints for 'assessments', practitioners using SFP will slow down and listen intently with constructive ears (Lipchik, 1988). Another variation in response to 'I don't know' could be, 'If our conversation today is a good use of your time, how might you know at the end?'. Throughout, we must carefully match our volume (quietened), tone (gentle) and pace (slow) with the client's circumstances.

SFP honours the client's struggle whilst endeavouring to co-construct the description of their desired outcome in their everyday life. We listen for the client's reasons for living and what keeps them 'on this side of life', amplifying these instead of trying to weaken or destroy reasons for dying (Fiske, 2008). Clients maintain their agency and control over an outcome other than suicide by hearing themselves talk about how they have managed to continue living (Froerer & Walker, 2023) rather than what is driving them to think of suicide (Fiske, 2017). We focus on client language without professional jargon or practitioner interpretations.

Safety-planning

Some organisations require a formal safety plan to be developed with anyone experiencing a suicidal crisis. SFP is inherently a safety-planning conversation.

Research currently underway (Leckning et al., 2023) is establishing that practitioners (compared to people with lived experience) are 'more likely' to view safety planning as beneficial and helpful in securing good outcomes, whereas people with lived experience find that during a crisis, safety-planning mainly helps them to avoid the need for hospital.

If offered, safety-planning needs to honour the client's agency and autonomy, particularly if the client has identified what works for them. Resources elicited from Solution Focused conversations are invaluable here. Some examples in my own practice have included: the knitting of a blanket one row per day, as an acknowledgement of being alive to do so; the keeping a photo of children on a phone wallpaper to remind someone of a reason for living; or listening to the loudest metal music (as enlivening in dark times).

Questions for co-constructing safety might include: how have you kept yourself safe in the past? How will you and others know that your confidence in keeping yourself safe is growing? (Iveson, 2018). Who is best placed to share your confidence about keeping yourself safe, and what works for you? These questions might contribute to the development of a safety plan by deriving practical information about safety milestones, including other person perspectives.

Documentation

SFP builds and amplifies safety whilst also being able to understand risk (thoughts, plans, intent). Multi-disciplinary conversation, as well as documentation of the conversation, are important requirements of many organizations. This is encouraged for all practitioners and can form part of Solution Focused work.

Anonymized case example

Louisa, 28 years old, is a woman we had been asked to 'assess' for short-term (Crisis Team) support. She was due to go home from an intensive care unit after surviving a suicide attempt by overdose. I read a brief synopsis about her before we met, my best hope being to have a genuine, hopeful, Solution Focused conversation and to trust the SFP process. Louisa had been assessed daily whilst in hospital by the Liaison team.

'P' stands for practitioner. 'L' is Louisa, the client.

P: Hi Louisa (*introduced self and colleague*). What are your best hopes from us talking today?

L: No one has ever asked me a question like that. I don't know. (*Pause while I waited for her to think a little longer and find an answer*). Do you know who I am? I'm one of the naughty ones. I used to be in the ED like 40 times a year! I've tried to kill myself so many times . . .

P: We haven't met before. Forty times a year? And yet I noticed you haven't been here for the past four years?

L: Yeah, I haven't been here as a patient for years.

P: Given that it's been years, how will you know us talking has been a good use of your time? (*A best hopes question*).

L: I don't know. I don't want to end up like I was over four years ago.

P: What would you like to see happening instead?

L: I want to get back to work soon, maybe next week. Start seeing my therapist again. Be around for my son.

P: And if you could get back to work, see your therapist again and be around for your son, what impact are you hoping that might have for you?

L: I don't know. You ask hard questions. (*P nods and waits*). I wouldn't be worried about work so much and things whirling around in my head.

P: Instead of worrying about work and things whirling around in your head, what might you notice?

L: I would feel **more content and OK with my life, like, just be in the moment and maybe enjoy some things.** (*Best hopes and desired outcome verbalized*).

P: If we could spend time talking about you being more content and OK with life, just be in the moment, maybe enjoy some things, would that be OK for you?

L: Yes.

(Already my Solution Focused 'hearing' was noting so many resources spoken by Louisa: she had a number of best hopes; had been living her life without mental health service contact; had recognized that seeing her previous therapist might make a difference; she wants to be around for her son; and she explains that this had led to significant change four years ago).

P: Thinking back over past years, when was a time you felt content and OK with life, having enjoyed something? Even just briefly?

(An opportunity to hear about hope and living. Presupposing Louisa had done something different to avoid attending an ED in our area. Hearing about her life in the past four years would allow me to listen for more resources, qualities and skills).

L: When I got into my course.

(We begin to hear the history of the outcome she was hoping for).

P: And thinking back, when you were doing your course and OK with life in the past, perhaps in the moment and maybe having enjoyed something, how did you manage to get from being a client here four years ago to studying and working? (Asking from a not-knowing stance with genuine belief and awe that she has managed this herself).*

L: I kept being put in hospital when I attempted suicide or cut myself. I've tried to kill myself so many times, probably 50. They were going to put me in the long-term locked ward. When I heard that, I just thought, 'Nope, I won't let them do that to me'. Didn't want to let that happen. Wanted to be around for my son – not locked up.

P: How did you 'not let it happen'; not get locked up?

L: I told my therapist back then, I wanted to study, to do something, so I enrolled in a course. I was sick of what happened to me when I was a kid, playing over and over in my head.

P: And at that time, how did you know that studying was the right thing for you?

L: I just knew I wanted to do something to help people 'cause I was sick of people trying to help me.

P: And what difference did that make enrolling in the course? What course was it?

L: I enrolled in nursing. It felt good being able to do the course. Didn't like the book work so much, but really enjoyed my placements.

P: What qualities or skills did you draw on to be able to feel good, to do the course, even though you didn't like the book work, but you enjoyed the placements?

L: I suppose I was pretty determined not to get locked up and be around for my son, to be his mum.

P: Determined, you were determined. What's your son's name? How old is he?

L: Sonny is six years old. Lives with my mum because I'm still trying to increase my time with him.

P: Sonny stays with you sometimes?

L: Yeah, three nights a week, and depending on my shifts, I either take him to school or pick him up. I live with his dad. We're not together, just live in the same house. Don't really like his dad. We're housemates only.

P: Even though you don't particularly like Sonny's dad, how do you manage to continue living there?

L: It's somewhere for Sonny to stay when he is with me. I need somewhere for him to be with me and that's all I can afford.

P: So having somewhere for him to stay during his time with you sounds important.

L: Yeah, of course it is. I haven't been much of a mum to him since he was born. Mum's had him most of the time.

P: And even though your mum's had him most of the time . . . . When you have been the mum you have wanted to be, what things have pleased you the most?

L: He's with Mum because Children's Services said he couldn't be with me full time back when I was so bad going to ED all the time.

P: OK, and since then, you mentioned you now have him three nights a week and do school drop off and pick up. What pleased you the most since the early days?

L: I don't know (long pause, I remained silent, giving her time to think). I suppose I used to do drugs a lot, like anything you can think of, and I stopped it all about three years ago. All except cigarettes. I only stopped them about a year ago.

P: You stopped using drugs three years ago and cigarettes about a year ago. What impact did that have?

L: Well, stopping the drugs meant I didn't have to do the urine screens for Children's Services after a year of clean screens, and I got to be with Sonny more.

P: You got to be with Sonny more. How did you get to that point?

L: I just thought, if I didn't work out a better way of doing things, I wouldn't see him again. He's my son. I wanted to be his mum more.

P: What else did you notice about yourself, leading to you being his mum more?

L: I felt good knowing I could finish my course and start working, and, in between, make time to be his mum. Like the school drop-off and pick-up, sleepovers and be there more for him.

P: What difference did that make, feeling good knowing you could be there more as his mum?

L: I don't know . . . I just love being his mum. (Reason for living).

P: If we were to ask Sonny what he noticed about you that tells him you love being his mum what might he say? (Interactional questions bringing the description into reality).

L: He knows I love him. I tell him and cuddle him lots.

P: And what is it about the way you tell him and cuddle him that tells him you love him?

L: Give him a cuddle whenever I see him. I tell him, 'Mummy loves you so much. Do you know how much? To the moon and back!'

P: And how does he respond?

L: He cuddles me back and says, 'And I love you to the moon and back too'.

P: And are you pleased?

L: Yes.

P: How would he know that it pleases you?

L: I smile and tickle him, and we laugh together.

P: So, being the determined Louisa who wants to do the nursing course and be around for her son . . . what other qualities or skills did you draw on?

In the rich description of her recalling the time of being 'content and OK with life, in the moment and enjoying life', I could hear hope building. This part of the conversation gathered the 'history of the outcome' *and* a 'history of her resources'. All through this conversation, Louisa heard herself speak this information aloud. There were no suggestions or cheerleading from me, just the next question in response to her last, keeping her actual words integral to the questions and the desired outcome in mind.

This description (about 15 minutes of talking) was gathered without me having to ask a single problem-oriented question. I had no intention of removing the problem(s), and yet her description from our co-constructed conversation gave me an insight into the version of herself that she wanted to be, most of which had already been present in her life. Parts of that description included her letting me know about the many obstacles and challenges that she had navigated. Some of these included finding ways to survive childhood sexual abuse and a difficult relationship with her son's father, to live relatively substance-free for three years and tobacco-free for almost 12 months.

At this point, she exclaimed, 'Gee, I've come a long way, haven't I?'. I replied, 'Yes, it sounds like you *have*' (no cheerleading, simply acknowledging she has come a long way). Louisa then said quietly, 'I just wish what he did to me when I was a kid didn't affect me when I feel stressed' (*She was referring to childhood sexual abuse*).

I acknowledged, quietly and slowly, the impact that must have had on her life over many years. Then I tentatively offered: 'It sounds like the past interferes with your life sometimes'. She agreed and said she 'wished it could be different'. I went on to ask, 'If it could be different, what might be the first small sign that your past is no longer interfering with your future?'

Louisa paused, then said, 'I've never thought of it that way. I need to think about this . . .'. After a pause of 20 seconds (which made my non-Solution Focused colleague shift in their seat), Louisa told me the first small sign: that she wouldn't feel powerless or hopeless at her new workplace if she didn't know something. 'And instead?' I asked. She would 'work it out and have the courage to ask for help from someone, then get on with doing' what she needed to do. I asked, 'What difference might that make?' And the co-construction of this part of her preferred future began, incorporating her resources and the history of the outcome.

I asked if we could go back a few steps to what she might notice the next morning if 'this is the day the version of her, content and OK with life, in the moment and enjoying life, with the courage to ask for help at work, might be present?'. What might be the first small sign that would tell her? And what time might it be? (*Creating the scene of time and place in the future*). And what else?

Each question was constructed in response to her last, using her language, asked from a not-knowing stance and with the belief that she has and will be able to be 'content and OK with life: in the moment and enjoying life'. As her description of the small signs grew, I checked who she might see first. She mentioned her mother and Sonny. Interactional questions followed. What might they notice that tells them this version of her is present? How would she know they noticed? How would *they* know she knew? These interactional questions, whilst highlighting her connection to others, also embedded the co-constructed future into her important relationships.

Given that she was talking about her son and mother again, I asked her: 'If we were to make something like a list . . . perhaps called reasons for living . . . where might your son and your mother be on that list? And who or what else might be on that list?'

This conversation was full of Louisa, her language, her resources and her preferred future, with an abundance of examples of how she planned to keep herself safe as she moved into that future.

Louisa was offered the opportunity to write a formal 'How I keep myself safe' plan; however, she said that, for now, she knew what she wanted to do. She planned to call her previous therapist the next day when she woke up. She basically summarized our whole conversation about the next day, including multiple examples of her growing safer in the future. The conversation provided enough information for my non-Solution Focused colleague to write the organizational risk assessment and plan.

Louisa was agreeable to seeing the Crisis Team for a few days whilst she re-connected with her therapist. This agreed plan included our next colleague to see her asking, 'What has been better since the last meeting?'

References

Blundo, R., Bolton, K., & Hall, C. (2014). Hope: Research and theory in relation to solution-focused practice and training. *International Journal of Solution-Focused Practices*, 2(2), 52–62. https://doi.org/10.14335/ijsfp.v2i2.22.

Connie, E. E., & Froerer, A. (2023). *The solution focused brief therapy Diamond*. Hay House Inc.

Fiske, H. (2008). *Hope in action – Solution focused conversations about suicide*. Routledge Taylor and Frances.

Fiske, H. (2017). Solution-focused brief therapy and suicide prevention. *International Journal of Brief Therapy and Family Science, 7(1)*, 1–2. https://doi.org/10.35783/ijbf.7.1_1.

Froerer, A., & Walker, C. (2023, September). Solution Focused Universe monthly content. *SFBT and Suicidality* (video). Retrieved September 1, 2024, from https://members.solutionfocusedbrieftherapy.com/course?c=MjAyMzA5&lid=NTMx

Iveson, C. (2018, March 20). *Solution focus and risk.* www.brief.org.uk/blog/2018/03/20/solution-focus-and-risk/

Leckning, B., Shand, F., Proctor, N., Martin, A., Ferguson, M., & McGill, K. (2023). *Australian experiences with suicide safety planning* [Summary of Research Project]. www.blackdoginstitute.org.au/research-projects/australian-experiences-with-safety-planning/

Lee, M. Y. (2003). A solution-focused approach to cross-cultural clinical social work practice: Utilizing cultural strengths. *Families in Society, 84(3)*. https://doi.org/10.1606/1044-3894.118.

Lipchik, E. (1988). *Interviewing with a constructive ear* [Online Post]. Dulwich Centre Newsletter.

Ratner, H., George, E., & Iveson, C. (2012). *Solution focused brief therapy – 101 Key points and techniques* (1st ed.), Routledge, Taylor and Frances Group.

Shand, F., Vogl, L., & Robinson, J. (2018). Improving patient care after a suicide attempt. *Australasian Psychiatry, 26(2)*, 145–148. https://doi.org/10.1177/1039856218758560

Wright, P., Badesha, J., & Schepp, G. K. (2015). Balancing a solution-focused approach with traditional psychiatric assessment in a Canadian emergency room. *Journal of Systemic Therapies, 33(4)*, 24–34.

Chapter 13

Helping AMHPs to be AMHPs – Solution Focused Practice under the Mental Health Act 1983 (as further amended)

Nick Perry

In their article published in 2018, Minna Sadeniemi and team helped us to begin to understand the scope of, and differences between, the systems and processes for supporting and treating citizens with mental ill-health across Northern and Southern Europe.

Mental health systems across Europe and across other continents may or may not have statutory roles similar to that of the Approved Mental Health Professional (AMHP) in England and Wales (Mental Health Act, 2007).

AMHPs can have professional training backgrounds in social work, nursing, occupational therapy and psychology but are not permitted to be doctors. In my article with David Watson, published in 2022 on *Solution Focused Practice and the role of the AMHP,* we recall that:

The AMHP intervenes in a crisis, where there may be muddle and confusion, as well as a state of panic (Parkinson & Thompson, 1998). Leah (2020) describes the AMHP as having a hybrid role, including as mediator, advocate, custodian of social justice and – of relevance to this article – therapist.

But as Jill Hemmington (2023) has argued, and in the context of increasing pressure on National Health Service (NHS) resources in the UK (BMA, 2023), there is increasing uncertainty within the AMHP workforce about what, and who, AMHPs are for?

As written into the Mental Health Act 1983 (as amended in 2007 and soon to be further amended), AMHPs have a duty to consider a client's situation for their employing local government authority (Section 13) and, if the legal grounds are met – and there is no safe, less restrictive option available – to make an application for compulsory admission for assessment or treatment.

There is a requirement to consider 'all the circumstances of the case' and where an application for compulsory admission is to be made, it must be based on the provision of two valid medical recommendations (where practicable, from a doctor with 'previous acquaintance' and also from a Section 12 'approved' doctor, with particular specialism in psychiatry).

What is becoming increasingly clear for the AMHP workforce is that despite the legislative changes and developments of four decades since the introduction of the Mental Health Act 1983, there has remained little or no guidance – and no

DOI: 10.4324/9781003519225-13

significant research base – as to how AMHPs should frame their interventions or convene their assessments (Hemmington, 2023; Blakley, 2023; Simpson, 2024).

The Code of Practice (Department of Health, 2015 also soon to be updated) – which is the main guidance document for AMHPs and other professionals involved in the statutory assessment process for people in mental health crises in England and Wales – has provided Guiding Principles for multi-disciplinary practice; and stipulates that time alone with an AMHP, for somebody being assessed under the Act, 'should usually be given' (14.54). But, there is no guidance as to how this client time should be structured or what skills are needed in order to make this time as useful as it could be.

This has been the context of my thinking and writing on this subject (Perry & Watson, 2022). And there have been parallel avenues of AMHP practice development over these post-pandemic years –perhaps signalling some morphic resonance in the AMHP world (Sheldrake, 2012). The work considers our duties and powers (Simpson, 2024; Mitchell et al., 2024); as well as the application of other therapeutic techniques, such as dialogical approaches, which Lauren Jerome references in her chapter, and which contain similarities to Solution Focused Practice (SFP) when applied to AMHP work (Manchester, 2022).

The principles of procedural justice, as Emma Burns has written about in Chapter 10, might also provide a framework for evaluating both the efficacy and the experience of AMHP work, just as they have done for policing, despite these roles being vastly different.

All this being said, what makes the Solution Focused (SF) approach such a good fit with the role of the AMHP is that it can be used in a one-off interview situation to good effect. As Guy Shennan has shown us in his chapter – it can be used to prioritise the voice of the client in a mental health crisis, moment by moment.

My own chapter contains two anonymised examples which demonstrate the use of SFP whilst undertaking the AMHP role. The first story seeks to explain something of how SFP, within 1:1 conversations, can support AMHPs to practice in anti-racist ways.

SF training and the format of my practice stories

In learning to become a Solution Focused practitioner, I have benefited from reading transcripts of SF conversations that teachers and trainee colleagues have had with their clients. I have seen videos, and I have spent time thinking about and practicing how to ask SF questions. This has begun to teach me – experientially – how to build a subsequent question from the client's last answer. I have begun to be able to keep the client's focus on what we might have agreed as their best hopes (our loose contract for working together), perhaps with the development of some detail about their preferred future; perhaps with a scaling question or two along the way.

The application of this training and learning to my statutory role – assessing children and adults in mental health crises and working out (with their help and collaboration) the least restrictive support plan which can make things better for them – has been an important development in my professional life. There has been no advanced, AMHP-specific training on how to do this; it is a journey that I have undertaken largely on my own, and in some ways, it has been one of the key motivating factors encouraging me to write (and campaign) about the impact of SFP on, and the obvious benefits for, AMHP practice (Perry, 2023; Samuel, 2023).

I have made a decision that the anonymised practice stories included in this chapter will be provided in the format and in the formal reporting style that I have developed as an AMHP. This is in order that AMHPs who are reading will be able to relate to the practice situations that I have found myself in, that I will be speaking their professional language and that I will be able to demonstrate how I have been able to 'twin-track' my interventions. This is a phrase that I have learnt from Evan George and indicates the duality of a statutory role and function alongside the possibility of a therapeutic intervention.

First is the story of Rohan. This was an assessment that I undertook in early 2022 (during a period when we were still wearing face masks due to the pandemic). I was three months into a year-long advanced certificate in SFP with BRIEF (George et al., 2013).

Excerpts from the anonymised report are provided in what follows. I first met Rohan – a young, British man of mixed heritage (White British and Black African) in his late twenties – after he had been arrested for an assault on his younger brother in the family home (he had been visiting; he lives in a different city):

There was no opportunity for the AMHP to meet with the client ahead of the assessment because of the time between referral and co-assessor availability, but also because of the level of agitation that the client was experiencing.

During the initial brief phase of the interview, where the AMHP and Dr Dani were attempting to ascertain whether or not the client could be interviewed in the interview room of the Custody Suite rather than his cell, he was standing and shouting in a hostile manner. He was presenting as paranoid and grandiose. He was understandably unhappy about having been held in the Police Station since the previous evening, and it did not feel safe to the assessors to move him from the cell due to the unpredictability of his behaviour.

[Given his presentation, Police colleagues had recommended that Rohan be assessed in his cell]

He seemed to notice that he was being assessed by a person of colour, so the AMHP and Dr Dani took the main roles in the assessment, with Dr Norman being party to the interview out of the view of the client by the door of the cell.

According to the officers who handed over information to the assessors, Rohan has been talking to himself whilst in his cell. Although he was not obviously responding to any psychotic experiences during the interview that was had in his cell, his mood was highly changeable and he went from shouting at the AMHP to talking calmly in a very short space of time.

Rohan made comments about Dr Dani smiling behind his mask and the AMHP speaking in a 'patronising' voice in a way that suggested a degree of persecutory ideation. There [were] no suicidal thoughts evident and no obvious intent to be physically aggressive, but Rohan was angry and he made that clear to the assessors.

It was not easy to assess his mood in full; however, he had energy, and it did not seem as though he was depressed.

Offered some sedating medication (following advice from the assessing doctors) by the custody nurse, he declined the medication, saying that he did not trust the professionals who had been speaking with him.

As a result of this brief interview, the circumstances of arrest, the levels of agitation and the lability of Rohan's mood, the two assessing doctors were minded to make medical recommendations for a section 2 detention (compulsory admission to hospital for assessment followed by treatment) – on the basis that he was thought to have a mental disorder of a nature or degree which warranted the same; there were risks evident to others; and that there was no (safe) less restrictive way of providing the support that he needed.

When arranging any medical examinations, the AMHP is at liberty to choose the assessing doctors. In this case, I had chosen two male psychiatrists, one with a forensic specialism. One doctor was White British; one was Indian. There was no possibility of having a doctor present who had 'previous acquaintance' as Rohan had been visiting from out of the area.

Whilst the doctors were able to make their medical recommendations, I (as the AMHP) was not in a position to make an application for compulsory admission because a psychiatric bed had not been identified for Rohan.

This was despite one of the assessing doctors (the doctor of colour) making a clear recommendation to the Mental Health Trust that the client was suitable for an open ward and did not need to be admitted to a Psychiatric Intensive Care Unit (PICU). He had been judged (on the information describing his arrest) to be too risky for the available open ward, and the service manager of the unit (a White female) had declined to accept him. He was also declined by a PICU screening process for exactly the reasons that the assessing doctor had given in support of his appropriateness for an open ward. This ended up being raised as a matter of complaint by me, with Mental Health Trust and local authority managers on call.

As a result of these disagreements, the 24-hour period for which Rohan was permitted to stay in police custody (after arrest, under police legislation) came to an end, and he was placed under section 136. This is a police holding power under the Mental Health Act and carries with it an obligation for further specialist assessment of a client's mental health in a 'place of safety'. The situation for Rohan was helped at this point by a senior nurse (of colour) – as the result of a telephone conversation between us – agreeing to accept the client to a Health-based Place of Safety (HBPOS). The section 136 holding power is also for a 24-hour duration. It was in the HBPOS that I went to see Rohan again:

The AMHP has visited Rohan at the Place of Safety this afternoon further to confirmation from the Trust that a PICU referral will not be required and that, should there have been a need for it, there would [now] be a bed available locally at the inpatient unit; the AMHP has been able to update Rohan's mum Gina throughout yesterday evening and fielded a phone call from her early this morning regarding where her son has been taken; the AMHP was able to ask some Solution Focused questions and Rohan was willing to engage with the process which lasted over an hour – Rohan was much calmer in demeanour and he apologised for the way that he spoke to the assessors in the Police Station.

During the period of discussion, Rohan recounted how he experienced racism on a daily basis growing up and had a very difficult relationship with local police; he says this is part of the reason for his presentation in the cells on Tuesday afternoon.

Rohan was willing to explain what had led up to the 'explosion' on Monday evening: he had returned at the weekend after not having been at his mother's home for a long time (he said a year or year and a half); he said that he was not welcomed when he arrived; he says that he has helped try to make inroads into the condition of the house and garden over the weekend (for example he cleaned the bathroom and attempted to sort the garden by putting wood, metal and bottles into piles); Rohan explained that his mother had not been pleased with his efforts and he went out for a ride on his bike in order to avoid a disagreement. When he returned, he waited for a long time to be let in to the house. He then had an altercation with his brother. He said that he does not remember how this started, although his brother will have been tired from his work (with a scaffolding firm). Rohan describes smashing photo frames and taking the pictures of himself because he feels as though he is a 'trophy family member' without any real relationship with his mother and brother. During the conversation, Rohan spoke about his mother's mental health needs and the role he took on in his younger life, providing a level of care for her. He says that he has seen things that he should not have seen as a child. He says that he thinks his mother holds some guilt for this.

Rohan acknowledged during the conversation that he may benefit from some psychological support in order to build a future that suits him. He contracted to re-register with a GP in Oxford when he gets home and to seek out the possibility of some counselling. Due to having spent an extended period in Custody and then having been detained under section 136 of the MHA 1983, Rohan was not keen to accept the AMHP's offer of a further night in hospital as a voluntary patient. He has accepted a taxi journey to [the nearest train station], where he will buy a train ticket to Oxford. Rohan has the keys to his father's home and says that there is food at home. He says that he has a nice neighbour who will help him, and he has been able to have supper (and take some snacks) from the Place of Safety.

It is the understanding of the AMHP that Rohan will not face any charges in respect of [the] incident and his arrest.

During the conversation, Rohan was future-focused, talking about trying to get work (although he realises that this may need to be unskilled work for a while and that he may find this boring). He was willing to answer a Solution Focused 'tomorrow question' in a detailed way, thinking about how life might be if relations with his mother and brother were at a point where they suited everyone.

He was willing to safety-plan regarding a return to home to collect some things before going back to Oxford. Rohan used the AMHP's phone to have a telephone call with his mother in the Place of Safety. During this time, the AMHP went to provide a verbal handover to the charge nurse to explain that an admission would not be necessary. The phone call did not go well, as far as Rohan was concerned, and so he has made a decision to return to Oxford directly, following the AMHP's decision not to make an application for section 2 detention.

The AMHP has phoned Rohan's mum, Gina, to inform her of the outcome of the assessment and Gina has been upset. She wanted her son detained to hospital. The AMHP has explained that during the period of interview, there were no positive symptoms of psychosis and the client did not present as experiencing anything unusual. His presentation at hospital has been totally different to that in Custody.

He has been reflexive; he was appropriately tearful at times, describing a long history of difficult family relationships; he is not presenting with any symptoms of depressive illness. He had a congruent and reactive affect; he has slept well at the [Place of Safety] and eaten appropriately. He is not suicidal; he has hopes for the future; he does not want to harm others and intends to stay away from his mother and brother for now.

The AMHP has discussed the interview with [the relevant] practice manager and has obtained an undertaking from Rohan to make contact via phone or email to confirm that he has arrived home safely.

The AMHP will update the [statutory report] with the information from to-day's interview. Charge nurse has been informed of his discharge from section 136 and the Place of Safety. He has been taken via the AMHP taxi account to the local train station.

Email feedback from Rohan later that evening:

Hi, just to let you know, I've arrived back in Oxford safe and sound. Thank you for treating my case so delicately and professionally. I know it's not been the best circumstances, but it was a real pleasure meeting you. I will be in further contact regarding the local GP and what they can provide for me up here. Please take care of yourself in the meantime, and I'll be in touch soon. Thanks again, Rohan.

What questions were asked; what difference did they make?

It is my firm belief that it was both the Solution Focused approach to the assessment as well as the Solution Focused questions asked that gave the opportunity for new information about Rohan's experience – in custody, of racism growing up and about his family – to be obtained.

It was then possible for me to balance the risk information which populated the referral for Mental Health Act work with this new information.

Whilst the content of the interaction is reported as a piece of section 13 consideration work which was inclusive of medical examinations (Mitchell et al., 2024; Perry, 2024a, 2024b), rather than as the transcript of a Solution Focused conversation, I remember the questions that I asked to have been classic Solution Focused questions. What are your best hopes for us talking together? And if we managed to achieve that, what difference might it make?

I was able to ask the tomorrow question and elicit information about what things would look like for Rohan, his brother and his mother if they were at 'a point where they suited everyone'. I remember vividly his describing the cooking of a breakfast for his brother: he had woken early and prepared a traditional meal, his brother had sat down, they ate together and they talked in a way that was helpful and healing.

Rohan was also able to talk about the future that he wanted in respect to work and his life in Oxford. He was able to speak in a way that demonstrated his cogency, and he demonstrated a level of calm and reflection that gave me the confidence to decline to detain him to hospital and instead prioritise his wishes: to let him go home to Oxford and obtain support from his local GP surgery.

The Solution Focused approach that I adopted married with my professional social work knowledge-base and anti-oppressive practice skills (Lee, 2003). The SF questions enabled Rohan to develop some confidence that I was genuinely interested in seeing his best hopes delivered and that I was able to practice in a way that took account of any worries he may have had or powerlessness he may have felt as a young British man of mixed heritage (Gajwani et al., 2016).

Although I did not do so on this occasion, there would have been nothing stopping me from using Solution Focused questions to frame my discussion with

Rohan's mum. Once I had introduced myself and explained the reason for my contact, I could have asked her what her best hopes were from our talking together – how she might have known that our talking together had been useful, both to her and to her son.

Perhaps the next case example – the anonymised report of my work with Selina – gives a better picture of how it might be possible to ask Solution Focused questions in a conversation preceding the involvement of section 12 doctors.

In my AMHP practice, I have found that it has been easier to ask Solution Focused questions in this 1:1 scenario (the time alone encouraged by the Code of Practice at 14.54) rather than in a multi-disciplinary interview. Having said this, being attuned to client capability and aware of problem-focused questions (which often derive the information for a psychiatrist's clinical impression) is also important when working alongside doctors. In my opinion, it is the role of the AMHP to chair these discussions in the best interests of the client.

As it happens, Selina's assessment took place a year later, in early 2023 (so, by this time, I was more practiced at applying SFP in Mental Health Act assessment situations).

Selina had also been detained under a police holding power (section 136) and had been taken to the local Emergency Department for an assessment:

The Approved Mental Health Professional (AMHP) has attended earlier to have the opportunity of [1:1 time with Selina] and to ask some Solution Focused questions. Selina was being supported by a male and female police officer in the family room at [the Emergency Department]. Police officer Mia was willing to stay in the room to support Selina in order to provide some gender balance.

AMHP has explained the process of assessment as Selina has not been detained under s136 before.

Asked what her best hopes for talking were, Selina did not know at first, but when asked how she might realise the conversation had been useful to her, she said that she might find herself starting to be happier. Initially, this was spoken of as finding herself 'happy all the time', but we settled on a loose contract of beginning to feel a 'normal amount of happy'.

Selina was willing to undertake the tomorrow question exercise and the AMHP was able to get some details about a preferred future.

Asked what would be the tiniest sign, when she woke up, that there had been a shift in her and that she was just a bit further forward toward being a normal amount of happy, Selina said that when she woke up, she wouldn't immediately reach out to people; she would find people reaching out to her.

On a school day, she would have woken up at about 7am, sprung out of bed with a bit of energy, made a cup of tea in a clean cup and sat in the conservatory.

The sun might be shining, there would be her music playing, and her morning tea would taste a bit sweeter.

Alex might have reached out and asked about her. He would have noticed the change in her by the tone of her voice and more positivity in the content of what she talked about. Selina spoke about Alex as a positive influence in her life and the lives of their children. Asked what Alex might say that he liked about Selina, Selina thought he might say her personality, her quirkiness and her smile. He appreciates her – they appreciate each other.

Selina lives with her younger daughters, Molly and Anna (12 and 5) – Anna would be the first of her daughters to notice this shift in her mum – she would notice her mum being happier and smiling; they would hug and they would both notice the different quality of this hug. It might lead to a gentler morning between them before going to school. Molly would also notice and maybe tease her mum a bit because she has a good sense of humour. Both children would be pleased for their mum, and her being happier and softer with them might lead them to spend more time talking with Selina.

This shift in Selina might well affect the journey to school – Molly goes to school by herself, but Selina regularly takes Anna on the bus. People on the bus who see her regularly might notice her wearing make-up and dressing a bit differently – her self-care being better; and that she would talk to them (whereas previously, she might not have spoken).

This imagined change – towards feeling a more normal amount of happy – might show up in Selina's posts on social media, which might end up being more positive in outlook. If Selina was feeling better, she might find herself posting inspirational quotes.

It would also show up in her being able to be more assertive, choosing to have more positive people in her life and not putting herself in dangerous situations (like the incident yesterday or with drugs). Instead, Selina might find herself having more time for her children and maybe going out with them (and the dog) to the beach.

Friends would notice the shift in Selina – Maria and Leona would notice the fact that she would meet them in town (probably at The Clarion for a drink and a baked potato). These are good friends of Selina's who would notice her more positive outlook. Maria always tells Selina that she doesn't want her to stop being the person that she is – she values Selina's quirkiness, directness and trustworthiness. Leona is also complimentary about Selina's style and the ways she has her hair.

Asked to score herself in relation to this imagined version of herself, where 10 is the day as imagined and 0 is the worst of times, Selina scored herself at 0. Asked how she had managed to keep going and not give up on herself when times had been tough, Selina worked hard to think about what had helped – she said the interest that Rob had shown in her had helped; also, the new puppy and getting out of the house had helped.

Asked how she would know that she had arrived one point up the scale, Selina said that she would find herself eating better, cooking fresh food for herself, improving her self-care and dress and that her house would be tidier. The children would definitely notice this change and would see their mum not moping about so much. Selina would be pleased with this, as would the children.

Asked later on how she would know that she was still going in the right direction even if there were future setbacks, Selina said that she would not turn to Rob and to drugs – these would be the key indicators for her.

The AMHP then took a break and advised Selina that the doctors would be coming shortly. When the doctors arrived, the [medical examinations] took place in the Liaison Psychiatry interview room. Police officer Mia remained [as a support].

The doctors established more detail about the past few days and the events leading up to the contact with the police and the s136 detention.

Selina has used cocaine on a daily basis during the three years following her father's death in 2019. On Friday, she returned from spending time with Rob in Bournemouth, where she had used Crystal Meth and Crack, and she started to feel suicidal on the train home . . . She ended up using a further gram of cocaine on Saturday and then took a decision to take a taxi to Warren Hill, where she said some goodbyes to friends and Maria called for police assistance.

In relation to her current risk of suicide, Selina scores herself at 6 (where the intensity of suicidal thinking was 10 yesterday). Selina believes that she needs some structure to her day to start reducing that score. She does not believe hospital admission will help her. She is open to support from the local Crisis Team (to whom she has been referred before) and the assessors have made this referral. She is also open to exploring specialist support from [a local service] regarding her cocaine use. Selina is aware that her drug use will have a negative effect on the efficacy of her prescribed medication. Some information was given in an interview about the positive effect of some stimulant drugs when there are ADHD symptoms, but there are come-down problems related to this and these appear to be difficult for Selina to cope with when she is in a vulnerable situation in her life. She mentioned that alongside the difficulties with Rob, she also has stress from money and housing worries.

Selina said she is interested in reading and cooking family meals, and these activities could give additional structure to her days. She is aware that [the Crisis Team] will contact her to make an assessment appointment.

The doctors have decided not to make any medical recommendations for hospital admission, and Selina has been taken home by police officers; the s136

detention is ended and [the Crisis Team] will follow up to provide interim intensive support as well as medication review. They will then likely hand back to the
longer-term treatment team at Cornwall House.

Selina has been encouraged to do some reading around different models of
therapy and explore which therapies could be helpful to her. She is aware that
EUPD can sometimes be helped by therapeutic interventions.

I hope that the reporting of Selina's assessment gives a fuller and richer demonstra-
tion of how a classic SF conversation structure (George et al., 2013) might assist
an AMHP in considering a client's case under section 13(1).

The classic opening question for a second session of SFP is often 'What has
been better?'. These case examples did not provide for a second session, as is often
the case in AMHP work, but such a question might well be useful to an AMHP
asked to consider the renewal of a Community Treatment Order (section 17A).

At the time of writing, neither Rohan nor Selina have re-presented for assessment under the Mental Health Act in our area.

Whilst it is not possible to know it as a matter of fact, it is the key contention
of this chapter that SFP has had a material impact for the better on their situations
going forward and that this way of making a brief intervention is something that
could and should be used by AMHPs in England and Wales (and by any professionals worldwide who undertake similar functions) to improve both client outcomes
and also to increase job satisfaction.

References

Blakley, L. (2023). Truly listening to accounts of Mental Health Act assessments: Reflections on my practice. *British Journal of Social Work, 53*(7). https://doi.org/10.1080/0963
8237.2021.1922624.

British Medical Association. (2023). *An NHS under pressure.* www.bma.org.uk.

Department of Health. (2015). *Mental health act 1983: Code of practice.* The Stationary
Office. GOV.UK (www.gov.uk).

Gajwani, R., Parsons, H., Birchwood, M., & Singh, S. (2016). Ethnicity and detention: Are
Black and minority ethnic (BME) groups disproportionately detained under the Mental Health Act 2007? *Soc Psychiatry Psychiatr Epidemiol, 51*, 703–711. https://doi.
org/10.1007/s00127-016-1181-z.

George, E., Iveson, C., & Ratner, H. (2013). *Briefer: A solution focused practice manual.*
BRIEF

Hemmington, J. (2023). Approved mental health professionals' experiences of moral distress: 'Who are we for'? *British Journal of Social Work, 00*, 1–18. https://doi.org/10.1093/
bjsw/bcad258.

Leah, C. (2020). Approved mental health professionals: A jack of all trades? Hybrid professional roles within a mental health occupation. *Qualitative Social Work, 19*(5–6),
987–1006. https://doi.org/10.1177/1473325019873385.

Lee, M. Y. (2003). A solution-focused approach to cross-cultural clinical social work practice: Utilizing cultural strengths. *Families in Society, 84*(3). https://doi.org/10.1606/
1044–3894.118.

Manchester, R. (2022). *Could these be the key elements of dialogical mental health act interviewing?* www.the-critical-amhp.com/blog/blog-post-two-x437a.

Mental Health Act. (1983). *Mental Health Act 1983* (legislation.gov.uk).

Mitchell, J., Lewis, R., & Simpson, M. (2024). *MHA assessments and s13(1) MHA 1983: 'New' AMHP practices within existing law*. AMHP Leads Network – Resources Page (padlet.com).

Parkinson, C., & Thompson, P. (1998). Uncertainties, mysteries, doubts and approved social worker training. *Journal of Social Work Practice*, *12*(1), 57–64.

Perry, N. (2023). *Give AMHPs the therapeutic tools that they need to underpin least restrictive practice*. Community Care.

Perry, N. (2024a). *s13 Consideration and solution focused practice – the 'why' and the 'how'?* Blog Home (the-critical-amhp.com).

Perry, N. (2024b). *s13 Consideration and solution focused practice – further reflections on a very good fit*. Blog Home (the-critical-amhp.com).

Perry, N., & Watson, D. (2022). Solution-focused practice and the role of the approved mental health professional. *Ethics and Social Welfare*, *17, 2023*(3). https://doi.org/10.10 80/17496535.2022.2159294.

Sadeniemi, M. (2018). A comparison of mental health care systems in Northern and Southern Europe: A service mapping study. *International Journal of Environmental Research and Public Health*, *15*, 1133. https://doi.org/10.3390/ijerph15061133.

Samuel, M. (2023). *AMHPs lack time for 'extremely important' pre-assessment work with people in crisis, finds survey*. Community Care.

Sheldrake, R. (2012). *The presence of the past: Morphic resonance and the memory of nature*. Park Street Press.

Simpson, M. (2024). Changing gears and buying time: A study exploring AMHP practice following referral for a Mental Health Act assessment in England and Wales. *British Journal of Social Work*, *00*, 1–20. https://doi.org/10.1093/bjsw/bcad271.

Chapter 14

The wellbeing benefits of Solution Focused Practice for helping professionals

Aine Garvey

Practitioner wellbeing is an important area to focus on, given the impact it has on areas such as productivity, staff retention, compassion fatigue and, ultimately, client safety and care (Søvold et al., 2021). As Emma Burns has noted in her chapter, professionals who work with people in crisis and distress are at risk of post-traumatic stress. Healthcare workers, particularly mental healthcare workers, are also at higher risk of burnout than the general population (Johnson et al., 2018). While not ignoring the painful realities seen in this line of work, Solution Focused (SF) practitioners have described over and over again the inspiration they have gained from hearing about client resources, strengths and successes. A repeated theme in discussions is not only the positive difference practitioners have noticed for clients but also for themselves.

Potential for vicarious resilience and workplace wellbeing

Solution Focused Practice (SFP) has the potential to mitigate some of the challenges faced by practitioners when supporting clients in crisis. This allows practitioners to tap into opportunities for vicarious resilience (that is, the positive impact that practitioners experience as a result of observing the resilience of their clients in the face of adversity) whilst not ignoring the complex work demands and challenging work contexts. Pérez Lamadrid and Froerer (2022) found this to be the case in their study that measured the impact of training in Solution Focused Brief Therapy (SFBT) on vicarious resilience for Bolivian protective family service workers. This study reinforced the personal accounts that Froerer and colleagues (2018) described in their chapter about their experiences of vicarious resilience as a by-product of SFP. Froerer, Von Cziffra-Bergs, Kim and Connie describe some of the differences SFP has made to their own professional and personal lives. As well as vicarious resilience, the authors describe their experiences of vicarious hope, compassion satisfaction and vicarious gratitude as they were inspired by the resources of clients who have managed to cope with and work through difficult experiences. These accounts are often repeated at SF conferences, online events and meet-ups because they continue to edify and inspire.

DOI: 10.4324/9781003519225-14

A small but growing number of studies are available that describe the impact of SFP on workplace wellbeing (e.g., Medina & Beyebach, 2014b; Schwellnus et al., 2020; Seko et al., 2021; Simm et al., 2011; Smith, 2010; Smith, 2011; Smith & Macduff, 2017). Findings from a recent systematic review (Garvey et al., 2025) include improved emotional wellbeing as a result of changes to approaching work and in-work practices, a sense of alignment with personal and organisational values and improved working relationships with clients, colleagues and teams. These themes will be discussed further in this chapter alongside the personal accounts of various practitioners.

SFP and social constructivism

Underlying SFP is the emphasis on the collaborative learning that happens within a social context. This social constructivist way of thinking about the world assumes that reality and meaning is constructed through social and interactive processes (Lincoln et al., 2011). Language serves to construct reality rather than merely describing or representing it. When the Solution Focused practitioner is part of conversations that are co-constructed around hoped-for futures, resources and what is already helping, they have the opportunity to learn from futures that are full of possibilities and hope. In addition, this way of thinking assumes change is constant, and appreciating this uncertainty can be reassuring in an ever-changing and uncertain world.

Social *constructionism* also assumes that cultural reality affects the experience of each individual (McNamee et al., 2020). This philosophy highlights the importance of the Solution Focused practitioner's stance towards valuing clients' (as well as colleagues' clients') unique experiences and how they are understood within a social, cultural, economic and political context. It is a way of working which is effective for and respectful to individuals (and groups) with diverse values and cultural practices (Lee, 2003). As a practitioner colleague recently noted, 'I think what strikes me about the approach here is that the rights of people to make decisions about their care is respected and at the forefront of our approach'. On this basis, we can say that SFP has the potential to support anti-racist and culturally competent practice (Lee, 2003).

The impact of SFP on clinical work

As Evan George highlights in his chapter, belief and trust in the client lay the foundations of SFP. This belief and trust allows practitioners to let go of having to be the expert with all the answers or to take on all the responsibility to solve problems. This letting go allows the practitioner to collaborate more with clients around their hoped-for futures, their resources and what they are already doing to that fits with these hopes. It allows the practitioner to ask questions in the belief that the client has the capacity to change and to listen actively for evidence of this capacity. Subsequent benefits for clinicians have been described in findings by researchers such as Smith (2011) as the deriving of more flexibility and efficiency in work practices and a reduction in unnecessary referrals, as clinicians are able to listen and find out what clients want rather than prescribing interventions that might not fit with what they need.

A practice example here mirrors these findings. A colleague who had been incorporating SFP into her work for a number of years described to me the impact of asking the clients their best hopes and what they were doing already when history-taking.

'When I ask SF questions,[1] I find out that clients are, in different ways, already doing many of the things I might previously have recommended'. She noted, 'I saved so much time and energy by just asking them'. She also noted, 'I think I'm listening differently now though; I mean that I am actually listening to the answers and views that clients share and that their answers will guide our work'. This meant that she was now spending less time trying to come up with the answers. Instead, she came away from sessions inspired by the resources and expertise of clients, even in very challenging circumstances. She also explained that her note-taking was briefer and generally written within the session and using the client's own words. Instead of writing reports in professional jargon, she changed to collaborative report writing where the client's voice was central to the report:

> It's them that have to remember what to do, so if we use their own words, they're more likely to remember and there's less stress on me trying to come up with the answer . . . by asking clients what they are already doing and what they think might help, we can come up with plans that are client-centred and relevant, not professionally-driven . . . I feel like I'm actually making a difference rather than churning out reports that nobody reads.

Another colleague explained,

> I learned the concepts of working in partnership and the importance of being family centred in university and these concepts are repeated in lots of trainings and policy documents . . . but in hindsight, when I was saying I'll work in partnership with you, I meant that I'll say what needs to be done and you'll agree, it wasn't until I started [using SFP] that I realised what partnership actually was . . . [SFP] gave me the tools to actually do the partnering.

Improvements in listening and reflecting with clients as well as colleagues and wider teams have been noted by several researchers (e.g., Bowles et al., 2001; Eaton et al., 2010; Medina & Beyebach, 2014a; Schwellnus et al., 2020; Simm et al., 2011; Smith & Macduff, 2017). These changes have influenced staff in several ways. They have included better job satisfaction, increased self-efficacy and confidence and self-fulfilment (Simm et al., 2011; Smith, 2011; Seko et al., 2021). Others have noted increases in overall energy, enthusiasm and motivation in their job (Simm et al., 2011; Medina & Beyebach, 2014a). Eaton et al. (2010) describe the difference that SF has made in a small team. They describe how the team was 'more positive in general' and how SFP permeated to other parts of the organisation. For example, scaling questions helped to put things into perspective and were used to talk about progress in general or to notice progress for colleagues. Schwellnus et al. (2020) observe that training in Solution Focused coaching has taught clinicians more than just a set of tools to use with clients, but also a philosophy that fits with their personal values and has permeated into their personal, as well as work life. This, in turn, has been reported as 'freeing' and 'liberating' for some workers in their study. Medina and Beyebach (2014b) have also found lower burnout scores for child protection workers who have started using SFP.

The benefits of SFP for client relationships and clinical teams

Studies have also described the difference SFP has made in connections between clients, colleagues and within teams. Solution Focused practitioners describe having better relationships with clients as they let go of taking the expert role, having more respect and trust in clients and noticing a willingness to interact and listen more to clients and colleagues. Seko et al. (2021) note that collaborating with clients in a Solution Focused way helps to improve relationships, as practitioners listen for stories of strength and resources in the face of challenges. Research participants have also noted that SFP helps to improve communication within their teams with better team cohesion and better relationships with colleagues (Bowles et al., 2001; Medina & Beyebach, 2014a; Schwellnus et al., 2020; Seko et al., 2021). Improvements are also observed in teamwork and staff morale. Additionally, Medina and Beyebach (2014a) found that training in Solution Focused Practice enables more democratic ways of working within teams as well as facilitating improvements in team communication.

Solution Focused conversations and philosophy have expanded from the clinical space to wider teamworking, further supporting practitioners in the workplace. Numerous books such as those by Burns and Northcott (2022), Shennan (2019) and Iveson et al. (2012) explain how Solution Focused questions can be embedded into team meetings, supervision and coaching to support clinicians better.

Including questions in meetings such as, 'What has been better since our last meeting?' helps to focus conversations and help gain contributions from the whole team. As one colleague noted, 'We're already talking about the problems; what I like about our meetings now is that we can also focus on what is in our control, what we can *do*'. Including Solution Focused questions when collaborating with colleagues as well as talking about clients can also contribute to a healthier and happier work environment (Dierolf, 2014). As SFP tends to build cooperation and engagement with clients, so too can it build engagement and cooperation within teams (Medina & Beyebach, 2014a, 2014b).

A colleague describes the impact of adopting the BRIEF team's position of imagining that clients and colleagues are in the same room when talking about them and the difference this made. He has noticed multidisciplinary team meetings becoming more friendly and respectful as staff have changed the way they talk about each other and about clients. He says, 'so the way that we work now, I feel, is a much more authentic way of working for me and lovely that that's shared among the team'.

While the changes mentioned previously can improve workplace wellbeing, SFP is not a panacea. It cannot be a Band-Aid for some of the organisational barriers in place, such as reduced staffing and resources. Additionally, while SFP holds that there are many ways for clients to make changes in their lives, so, too, are there many other approaches that can support staff wellbeing.

Solution Focused Practice does not seek to deny that problems exist; this is important given the issues highlighted earlier. It can acknowledge *both* challenges *and* opportunities at the same time. For example, staff can experience vicarious trauma and vicarious resilience simultaneously (Pérez Lamadrid & Froer, 2022). Vicarious resilience is useful to focus on, given the far-reaching implications for the work, whilst not ignoring the real and enduring challenges faced in practice. Solution Focused practitioners have also noted challenges in implementing SFP in their work, especially within systems that are built on the medical model (Schwellnus et al., 2020; Smith, 2011).

Supports from the wider Solution Focused community or more locally with Solution Focused supervision has helped to counter these challenges. The ideas highlighted in the chapter by Rose McCabe and colleagues (particularly in the section 'Helping newly trained SF practitioners to embed the approach') are relevant for all SF practitioners, not only to enhance skills in SFP, but also for the wellbeing supports that these provide. Some of these supports will be discussed in the following paragraphs.

SFP and supervision

Thomas (2013) describes Solution Focused supervision as an effective model of supervision that identifies, develops and maintains practitioner competencies and skills. Building on the assumptions of SFP, it emphasises collaboration between supervisor and supervisee in emphasising success, what went well and what can be learned. Solution Focused supervision has been implemented individually, in peer groups and in wider teams. Adaptations such as the 10-minute talk described by Burns and Northcott (2022) can be implemented when time is limited. Medina and Beyebach (2014a) find that team atmosphere and mood are improved as a result of the use of Solution Focused supervision and training. They also note closer personal bonds and improved working relationships with wider teams while Koob (2002) finds that that Solution Focused supervision helps trainee self-efficacy.

The practice example that follows shows how SF questions have facilitated reflection on a complex piece of work and how the professional's answers have been reported back by email:

Thanks very much for coming to the peer reflection group this morning and for sharing some thoughts on a recent assessment that you have been pleased with. I asked you what you thought John (pseudonym) might say if I had asked what had pleased him about the way you had undertaken your [Approved Mental Health Professional] duties on the day of the assessment. You said that John might have described you as kind. You went on to talk about how you went to extra effort to involve his family and keep them informed about decisions and developments. Asked what particular actions John might have spoken about, you mentioned having visited him at his bedside, reassuring him about what was going to happen, engaging with him about his teddy bear and his games, respecting him and listening to him. When I asked you what the doctors might have appreciated about your input that day, you said they may have appreciated your punctuality, having information about the situation ahead of arriving, being given updated information by you prior to the interview starting, that you took charge of the assessment and asked important, open questions and that you processed their claims on time! I asked you to score your own performance on that day where 10 on the scale is you at your very best and 0 is a very bad day on the rota. You scored yourself at 7 initially, but after talking thought that it might actually have been an 8/10 assessment. You realised that things had gone well on the day with a bed already being available for John. You recalled that your score was based on your ability to explain things well to John's mum, that relations with the ward were helpful and collaborative and that the ward sorted out the transport requirements. You thought it could have been an even better assessment if you had been able to get a CAMHS specialist doctor to attend – you tried to arrange one, but there were none available at the time required. You had even thought about delaying the assessment for a day to see if this would facilitate such a doctor attending, but it could not.

SFP: simple but not easy

A recent discussion with an SF colleague supports the notion of SFP being simple but not easy and how small changes can lead to big differences.

There had been some thought about whether SF was more suitable for 'X presentation/client/family but not for Y'. Slowly, these assumptions started to fade away as we observed what worked and did more of it – and began to trust and believe in all clients. Thinking back, asking 'best hopes' [questions] appeared daunting at first as we were used to working from a very different paradigm where the clinician decided the direction of assessment and therapy. With practice, practice and more practice, it became easier to ask better questions based on client answers. Peer supervision and practice, additional SF training, managerial support, linking in with the wider SF community, more practice, additional reading in SF, videos from SF Practitioners such as BRIEF[2] and Solution Focused Universe[3] all helped.

Over time, the more Solution Focused conversations we had with clients, the more ripples we noticed with the wider team. Meetings started to no longer be about 'difficult' or 'tricky' clients and we had fewer issues around compliance or why clients were reluctant to attend or be discharged. Discussions often focused on appreciation of what clients were already doing and how the service could adapt given their needs and resources. At the same time, the challenges in working in an under-resourced system weren't ignored and remain topics for discussion.

Conclusions

In addition to supporting clients in mental health crises, SFP can also be a source of vicarious resilience and wellbeing for the helping professionals involved. This way of working is built on a profound trust in clients and an unshakeable belief in their capacity for positive change. Out of this trust and belief, conversations which describe hope-filled futures can lead to better client-practitioner relationships, can spill over into brighter ways of working with colleagues and can have encouraging impacts even further beyond. As my colleague said, small changes can lead to big differences.

Notes

1 See Chapter 7 for Rayya and Mark's sheet of SF questions and Chapter 4 for Guy's useful ideas. Different lists of SF questions are available in books such as Burns and Northcott (2022), Iveson et al. (2012) or Shennan (2019). Practitioners will often say that it is helpful to them to keep such a list of questions handy so that they can keep trying to use SFP incrementally.
2 www.brief.org.uk/resources/mini-presentations.html
3 https://thesfu.com/sfbt-moments/

References

Bowles, N., Mackintosh, C., & Torn, A. (2001). Nurses' communication skills: An evaluation of the impact of solution-focused communication training. *Journal of Advanced Nursing, 36*(3), 347–354. https://doi.org/10.1046/j.1365–2648.2001.01979.x.

Burns, K., & Northcott, S. (2022). *Working with solution focused brief therapy in healthcare settings: A practical guide.* Taylor & Francis.

Dierolf, K. (2014). *Solution-focused team coaching.* SolutionsAcademy Verlag.

Eaton, M., Kay, A., & Moon, H. (2010). The sustainably solution focused organisation. *InterAction, 2*(1), 112.

Froerer, A. S., Von Cziffra-Bergs, J., Kim, J. S., & Connie, E. E. (2018). 15. Vicarious resilience in Froerer. In A. S. et al. (Eds.), *Solution-focused brief therapy with clients managing Trauma.* Oxford University Press.

Garvey, A. Burke, J., & van Nieuwerburgh, C. (2025). *The impact of solution focused interventions on workplace wellbeing: A systematic review.* [Manuscript submitted for publication]

Iveson, C., George, E., & Ratner, H. (2012). Brief coaching: A solution focused approach. Routledge.

Johnson, J., Hall, L. H., Berzins, K., Baker, J., Melling, K., & Thompson, C. (2018). Mental healthcare staff well-being and burnout: A narrative review of trends, causes, implications, and recommendations for future interventions. *International Journal of Mental Health Nursing, 27(1):* 20–32. https://doi.org/10.1111/inm.12416.

Koob, J. (2002). The effects of solution-focused supervision on the perceived self-efficacy of therapists in training. *Clinical Supervisor, 21,* 161–183. https://doi.org/10.1300/J001v21n02_11.

Lee, M. Y. (2003). A solution-focused approach to cross-cultural clinical social work practice utilizing cultural strengths. *Families in Society, 84*(3), 385–395. https://doi.org/10.1606/1044–3894.118.

Lincoln, Y. S., Lynham, S. A., & Guba, E. G. (2011). Paradigmatic controversies, contradictions, and emerging confluences, revisited. In K. Denzin, & Y. Lincoln (Eds.), *The Sage handbook of qualitative research.* Sage.

McNamee, S., Gergen, M. M., Gergen, M., Camargo-Borges, C., & Rasera, E. F. (Eds.). (2020). *The Sage handbook of social constructionist practice.* Sage.

Medina, A., & Beyebach, M. (2014a). How do child protection workers and teams change during solution-focused supervision and training? A brief qualitative report. *International Journal of Solution-Focused Practices, 2*(1), 9–19. https://doi.org/10.14335/ijsfp.v2i1.17.

Medina, A., & Beyebach, M. (2014b). The impact of solution-focused training on professionals' beliefs, practices and burnout of child protection workers in Tenerife Island. *Child Care in Practice, 20*(1), 7–36. https://doi.org/10.1080/13575279.2013.847058.

Pérez Lamadrid, M., & Froerer, A. S. (2022). Solution focused brief therapy and vicarious resilience in Bolivian protective family services workers. *Journal of Solution Focused Practices, 6*(1), 4. https://digitalscholarship.unlv.edu/journalsfp/vol6/iss1/4.

Schwellnus, H., Seko, Y., King, G., Baldwin, P., & Servais, M. (2020). Solution-focused coaching in pediatric rehabilitation: Perceived therapist impact. *Physical & Occupational Therapy in Pediatrics, 40*(3), 263–278. https://doi.org/10.1080/01942638.2019.1675846.

Seko, Y., King, G., Keenan, S., Maxwell, J., Oh, A., & Curran, C. J. (2021). Perceived impacts of solution-focused coaching training for pediatric rehabilitation practitioners: A qualitative evaluation. *Physical & Occupational Therapy in Pediatrics, 41*(4), 340–354. https://doi.org/10.1080/01942638.2021.1872758.

Shennan, G. (2019). *Solution-focused practice: Effective communication to facilitate change* (2nd ed.). Bloomsbury Publishing.

Simm, R., Hastie, L., & Weymouth, E. (2011). Is training in solution-focused working useful to community matrons? *British Journal of Community Nursing, 16*(12), 598–603. https://doi.org/10.12968/bjcn.2011.16.12.598.

Smith, I. C. (2011). A qualitative investigation into the effects of brief training in solution-focused therapy in a social work team. *Psychology and Psychotherapy: Theory, Research and Practice, 84*(3), 335–348. https://doi.org/10.1111/j.2044–8341.2010.02000.x.

Smith, S. (2010). A preliminary analysis of narratives on the impact of training in solution-focused therapy expressed by students having completed a 6-month training course. *Journal of Psychiatric and Mental Health Nursing, 17*(2), 105–110. https://doi.org/10.1111/j.1365–2850.2009.01492.x.

Smith, S., & Macduff, C. (2017). A thematic analysis of the experience of UK mental health nurses who have trained in solution focused brief therapy. *Journal of Psychiatric and Mental Health Nursing, 24*(2–3), 105–113. https://doi.org/10.1111/jpm.12365.

Søvold L. E., Naslund, J. A., Kousoulis, A. A., Saxena, S., Qoronfleh, M. W., Grobler, C., & Münter, L. (2021). Prioritizing the mental health and well-being of healthcare workers: an urgent global public health priority. *Frontiers in Public Health*, *9*, 679397. https://doi.org/10.3389/fpubh.2021.679397.

Thomas, F. N. (2013). *Solution-focused supervision: A resource-oriented approach to developing clinical expertise*. Springer Science & Business Media.

Chapter 15

Some conclusions and some more best hopes

Nick Perry

By the time this book is published, we may already have an amended Mental Health Act to work to in England and Wales. From what practitioners have seen of government plans so far, changes to practice are intended to be phased in over a number of years.

The guiding principles of the amended legislation, pulled forward from the 2018 Independent Review[1] (chaired by Professor Simon Wessely) – choice and autonomy, least restriction, therapeutic benefit and the person as an individual – are all engaged by the core assumptions and the practice model of SFP in ways that I hope – now you have read this book – are obvious.

A newly amended Mental Health Act will form part of the UK government's health mission (and 10 Year Health Plan):[2] to build a health service fit for the future.

Evan George's chapter speaks to this mission and how the use of Solution Focused Practice is compatible with the shifts that the government envisages – moving from analogue to digital, from hospital to community and treatment to prevention (although Evan suggests that we should, in fact, shift from treatment to service). Evan points to the flexibility of SFP and how the approach can be, and is being, offered via new technologies. And Lauren Jerome encourages us that its research base is promising.

Notwithstanding the UK government's intended shift from hospital to community (which will need to be properly resourced) and the obvious importance of prevention (which will also need proper resourcing), this book has been focused on the relevance of Solution Focused Practice to and its usefulness in the work and environments of mental health crisis.

Whilst we must invest in a healthier and more functional NHS, which is rebuilt to optimise wellbeing, we will always have crisis work to undertake and we must have professionals who are appropriately equipped for it.[3]

For this to be achieved successfully, there must be a re-focusing on the training needs of helping professionals and the practice models that they use, particularly if minoritised groups are to receive more person-centred services and the statistics of compulsory admission are radically to change.

My hope is that policymakers, NHS and local authority leaders reading this book will take note of the recommendations from Rose McCabe and her team

DOI: 10.4324/9781003519225-15

and embrace a model of practice which – as Adam S. Froerer writes – ensures marginalised individuals aren't asked 'to accommodate to the dominant position or perspective'.

It is one of the main contentions of this book that Solution Focused Practice can provide a shared therapeutic language between practitioners from different professional backgrounds and add something of real value to the development of better, more co-produced care.

Rayya Ghul and Mark Kilbey's chapter is so significant in this context. Celebrating service users 'doing it for themselves' is something that mental health services could and should do so much more. This is entirely in keeping with NHS England's person-centred care framework and the expressed wishes of the Health Education England Patient Advisory Forum:

> We hope to be valued for what and who we are, no matter how broken we may seem from the outside. We want to be offered choice to maintain our independence, dignity and sense of self worth. The challenge for the NHS and all health and care providers is to develop a mindset, which will preserve our freedom to help ourselves in true partnership.[4]

I hope that the work of Take Off will be inspirational for people who have lived experience of mental ill-health (and repeated, well-intentioned interventions by mental health professionals that don't always help enough).

Similarly, I hope that Natasha Adams' and Luke Goldie-McSorley's work in these pages will inspire professional colleagues who have responsibility for the development of crisis support for our children and young people. I know that Natasha means it when she says that she wants people to make contact with her – and she provides her email address at the end of her chapter for that very reason.

As high-level discussions continue regarding how Police services, the NHS and local authorities best work together to support people in mental health crisis in England and Wales, I hope that Emma Burns' experience from New Zealand provides pause and food for thought. Her exposition of the principles of procedural justice and their application to frontline policing could not come at a better time (and they may well have relevance to AMHP practice, too).

I hope that my own, Michele's and Nektarios' chapters serve to stimulate a conversation within our own professional bodies as to how we can begin more systematically to apply Solution Focused Practice in statutory environments of crisis in the service of better, less restrictive client experiences. And that our colleagues will take heed of Aine Garvey's words about vicarious resilience, practitioner wellbeing and sustainability.

All this said, we are aware that there are gaps in our book. We do not have a chapter from a Solution Focused GP, and we know, for example, that there is recent work from Wales showing that primary care saw the highest incidence of self-harm presentations in young people compared to other settings.[5]

We do not have a chapter devoted to people with learning disabilities. We don't have a chapter looking at Solution Focused Practice with people experiencing dementia. Such people will experience mental health crises, too.

Whilst Kidge Burns and Sarah Northcott's work[6] is a valuable resource regarding the importance of verbal and non-verbal communication strategies (and the use of different senses to facilitate communication), there is more work that we need to do to show how SFP can be of use in a wider range of mental health crises which engage multiple complex needs.

From my own AMHP practice, I know that there have been certain scenarios where I have found it more challenging to use SFP in its purest form – one such example being with a young man who needed relay interpreters, as well as a British Sign Language (BSL) interpreter, to communicate with me. I realised very quickly once the assessment process had started that SFP questions do not readily lend themselves to the syntax of BSL and need to be adapted if they are to be used in mental health crisis situations. Yet we know that SFP is used all over the world in languages other than English, where the adaptation of questions to accommodate translation difficulties is commonplace. We can have confidence that, with determination, ways can always be found to use the approach.

As Guy Shennan has shown us, we can use SF questions moment by moment. SF questions practiced and practiced, interweaved by skilful practitioners into their daily work can de-escalate risk, can unlock new and crucial information and can help people being assessed to feel accepted and valued for who they are. These questions can support people towards safety and hope.

Those of us who work in environments of mental health crisis should all be trained to use them.

Notes

1   Independent Review of the Mental Health Act – GOV.UK
2   Change NHS: help build a health service fit for the future – GOV.UK
3   CentreforMH_CareBeyondBeds.pdf
4   Person-centred care | NHS England | Workforce, training and education
5   Self-harm presentation across healthcare settings by sex in young people: an e-cohort study using routinely collected linked healthcare data in Wales, UK | Archives of Disease in Childhood
6   Burns, K., & Northcott, S. (2023). *Solution-focused brief therapy in healthcare settings: A practical guide*. Routledge.

Index

For Product Safety Concerns and Information please contact our EU
representative GPSR@taylorandfrancis.com
Taylor & Francis Verlag GmbH, Kaufingerstraße 24, 80331 München, Germany

www.ingramcontent.com/pod-product-compliance
Lightning Source LLC
Chambersburg PA
CBHW050612280326
41932CB00016B/3014

9 781032 856476